RACE HORSES AT RISK

OVERNUTRITION

DRUGS

BREAKDOWNS

LENNART KROOK AND GEORGE A. MAYLIN

Published
by
The Authors
Ithaca, N.Y. 14850

Printed in the United States of America
The Sheridan Press
Fame Avenue
Hanover, Pennsylvania 17331

Published by
The Authors
Ithaca, New York 14850

Library of Congress No. 88-91458

ISBN 0-9621868-0-5.

RACE HORSES AT RISK

OVERNUTRITION

DRUGS

BREAKDOWNS

LENNART KROOK, D.V.M., PH.D.
Professor of Pathology
New York State College of Veterinary Medicine
Cornell University
Ithaca, NY 14853
and
Professor of Radiology
Cornell University Medical College
1300 York Avenue
New York, NY 10021

GEORGE A. MAYLIN, D.V.M., PH.D.
Associate Professor of Toxicology
and
Director, Equine Drug Testing and Research Program
New York State College of Veterinary Medicine
Cornell University
Ithaca, NY 14853

CONTENTS

I. INTRODUCTION

Why do so few horses bred for racing ever get to training? Why do so few horses trained for racing ever race? Why do so many horses race for only a few years? Why do so many horses break a bone during training or racing?

Fractures, the most dramatic end of a racing career or the cause of a failure in training, are widely believed to be traumatic. Traumatic means that an excessive external force acts or has acted on the bone in question. Bad track conditions, a term that has never been defined, are considered the major cause of breakdowns, including fractures.

We have published the results of a study, "Track condition and racing injuries in thoroughbred race horses" (1), and have found that the track condition has no influence on racing injuries. We have studied a great number of fractures in thoroughbred race horses suffering a fracture during a race (2) or during training. We have found that the fractures occur because of an underlying disease. In other words, the fractures are pathologic. We have reported our findings in a scientific journal, so the information is available to the scientific community. The information is not, however, readily available to those most concerned: those involved in horse breeding, training, and racing. The purpose of this book is to convey the scientific information to trainers, breeders, and all those involved in racing in popular terms. The origin and definition of these terms are given in the Vocabulary Section.

As an introductory case, we present the problem of a well-bred yearling thoroughbred colt. He had had some minor lameness problems which were diagnosed radiographically as cysts in both front pastern bones and soreness of the suspensory ligament. With restricted exercise and daily treatments of oral phenylbutazone, the colt was considered sound. He was started back with light workouts on the lunge line. While lunging, the groom heard a loud pop from the right front leg prior to the colt falling down.

The post-mortem examination revealed a spiral fracture of the shaft of the arm bone. The fracture started in the neck of the arm bone and extended down to the lower end of the shaft. On gross examination, there were no visible changes in the bone to explain the fracture.

Under the microscope, on the other hand, dramatic changes in the bone structure were detected.

The head of the arm bone, as all limb bones, develops from cartilage. Depending on the bone, cartilage is converted into bone at predetermined times. In this case, large areas of cartilage persisted at an age where they should long ago have been converted into bone (Fig. i).

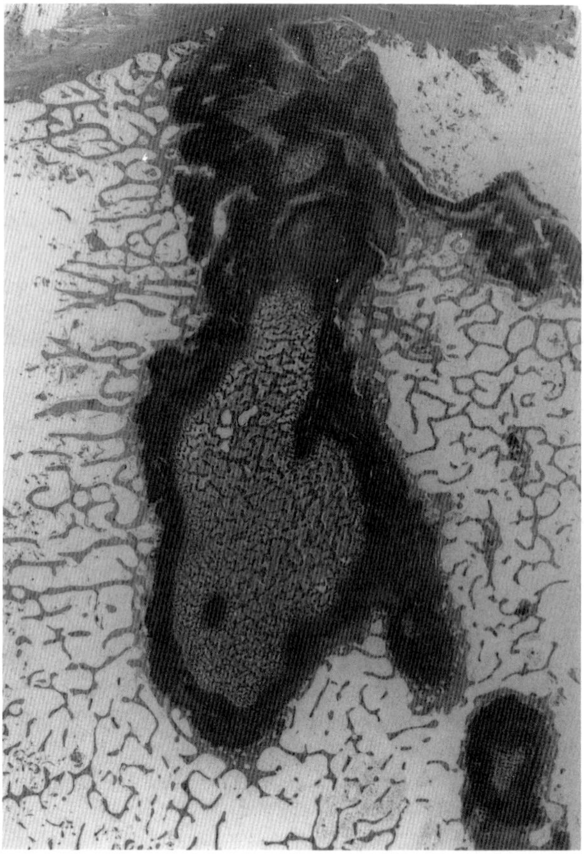

Fig. i. This is a microscopic picture of the head of the arm bone of a yearling thoroughbred colt. The inner part of the joint cartilage is at the top. The large black areas represent persisting cartilage which has failed to convert into bone.

In the growth area between the head and the shaft, the growth cartilage was very irregular and presented many cracks and separations (Fig. ii). The bone beneath the growth cartilage was more dense than normal. It was in this area of defective bone that the fracture started.

Radiographs of the front limbs from the fetlock joint and down showed a large cyst at the lower end of the left long pastern bone and one at the upper end of the right short pastern bone. A radiograph of a bone slice through the latter cysts appears in Fig. iii. Note that the cyst has no radiographic density, that the cyst is surrounded by dense bone and that it communicates with the joint surface by a soft channel. A microscopic section through this cyst is in Fig. iii. We will not go into

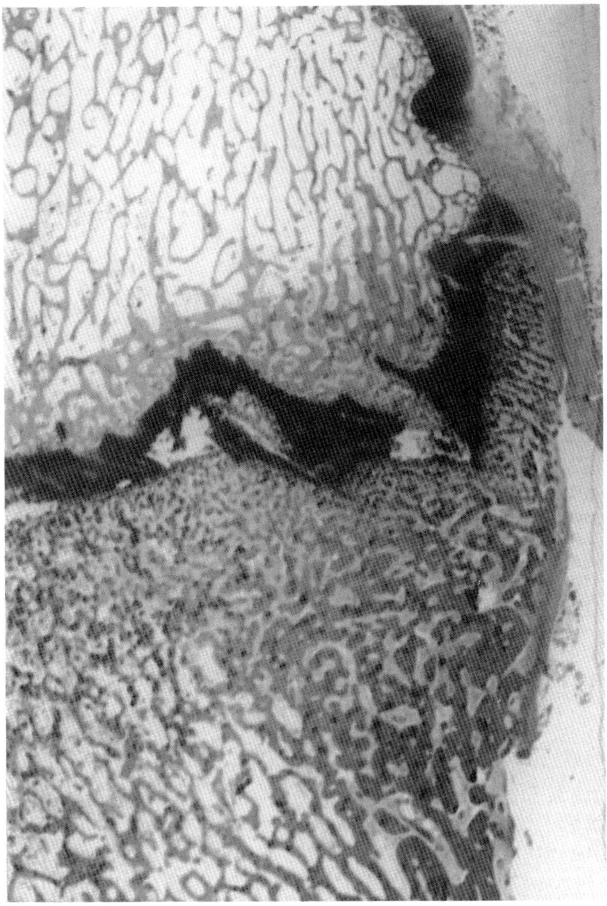

Fig. ii. Same colt as in Fig. i. The black horizontal band is the growth cartilage of the head of the arm bone. The band is irregular and presents wide cracks and gaps. The bone tissue beneath the plate is denser than normal. ×3.4.

the nature of the disease that caused this fracture and the cysts responsible for the lameness at this point—this will be appreciated by you after you have read this book. The pictures are presented here to show that the fracture and the lameness occurred because of existing disease and to underscore the importance of studying bones under the microscope. This is done by necessity—only to inform you, not to impress you.

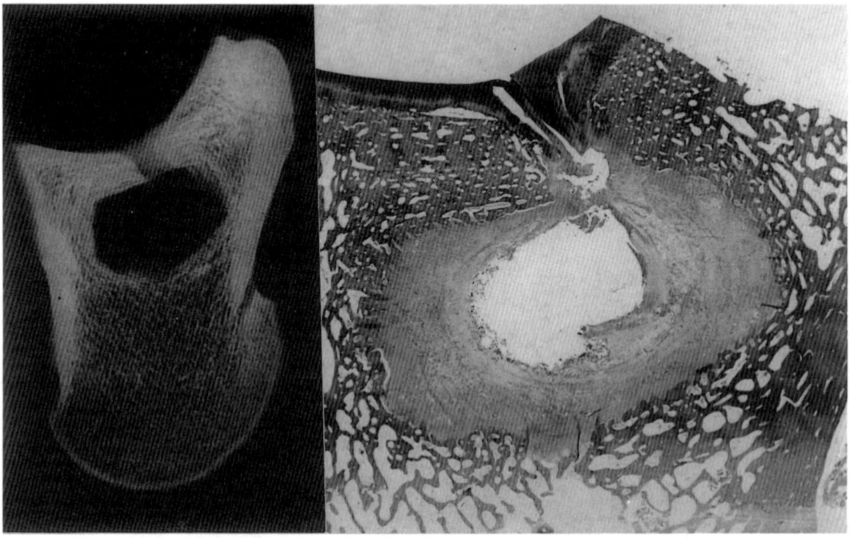

Fig. iii. Same colt as in Fig. i. To the left is a radiograph of a slab section through a cyst in the right front short pastern bone. There is a huge cyst in the upper end. The cyst has no radiographic density and is surrounded by dense bone. The cyst communicates with the joint surface by a soft channel.

To the right is a microscopic picture through the cyst, partly filled with dead cartilage. The surrounding bone is dense. The cyst communicates with the joint surface by a strand of cartilage. ×3.4.

A disease process is nothing fundamentally new to the body. Any disease process has its physiological or normal counterpart. Disease results when a biological process occurs at too little or too great an extent, at the wrong time, or at the wrong place. To understand disease, we must, therefore, understand the normal biological processes. In the case of skeletal disease in the horse, we must, accordingly, appreciate the normal development of the skeleton and the normal anatomy—gross as well as microscopic. We will include a description of the development of the horse skeleton beginning in the fetus and continuing in the growing foal. This will serve as a basis for understanding how disease of a limb occurs.

After describing skeletal development, we will provide a gross and microscopic description of breakdowns in horses. We will then give an analysis of data collected on track conditions how they relate or do not relate to breakdowns. We will, finally, propose the causes of breakdowns.

We will start our presentation with an illustrated description of the limbs of the horse. This will be straightforward anatomy of the gross appearance of the limbs.

REFERENCES

1. Hill, T., D. Carmichael, G. Maylin and L. Krook. 1986. Track condition and racing injuries in thoroughbred horses. Cornell Vet., *76:*361-379.
2. Krook, L., and G.A. Maylin. 1988. Fractures in Thoroughbred Race Horses. Cornell Vet., *78,* Suppl. 11. 1-133.

II. BONES OF THE LIMBS

In the preface to the second revised American edition of "An Atlas of Animal Anatomy for Artists" by W. Ellenberger, H. Baum and H. Dittrich, the Editor writes: "The quality of the Ellenberger plates is so fine that it has not been easy to find even a few more, strictly anatomical, studies from which could be made selections worthy to stand beside them." We agree. We tried to use photographs of anatomical specimens, but they did not match for instructive purposes the plates by Ellenberger, first published in 1901. So, we will go with the best and use them with permission of the publisher.

Fig. 1 is a drawing of a horse with a few skeletal landmarks indicated. A few more such landmarks appear in a superficial dissection (Fig. 2). The skeleton is shown in Fig. 3. From here on, we will be concerned with the legs only. First, a few terms. Memorize these terms as they will be used throughout the text.

Cranial Seen from in front; toward the skull.
Caudal Seen from behind; toward the tail.
Medial Seen from the midline of the body; inwards.
Lateral Seen from the outside; outwards.
Proximal In a limb—upwards.
Distal In a limb—downwards.

Bones of the forelimb

The forelimb is shown in cranial view in Figs. 4 and 5, in medial view in Fig. 5, in lateral view in Fig. 5 and in caudal view in Fig. 6. The bones of the forelimb are as follows:

Anatomical Name	*Popular Name*
Scapula	Shoulder blade
Humerus	Arm bone
Radius	Forearm bone
Ulna	Elbow bone
Carpus	Knee
Metacarpus III, MC III	Cannon bone
Metacarpus II and IV, MC II and MC IV	Splint bones
Proximal sesamoid bones	Sesamoid bones
1st phalanx, P I	Long pastern bone
2nd phalanx, P II	Short pastern bone

3rd phalanx, P III	Coffin bone
Distal sesamoid bone, navicular bone	Navicular bone

Sesamoid bones develop within tendons or joint capsules. They play or rub against other bones (articulate) and are able to withstand great pressure.

There are two sets of sesamoid bones in the forelimb of the horse. One pair, which is embedded in the suspensory ligament (definition to follow), is located on the back side of the lower end of the cannon bone. The other is the navicular bone, which is located at the back side of the joint of the short pastern bone and the coffin bone. We will use the term sesamoid bones to indicate only the pair of sesamoid bones associated with the cannon bone.

Figs. 1-6 also name some, but far from all, anatomical details of the front limb bones. Those named will be defined.

Lateral epicondyle of humerus. A condyle is a rounded projection of a bone that articulates with another. The lateral epicondyle of the humerus is located on the outside of the lower end of the arm bone.

Greater tubercle of humerus. Located on the outside of the arm bone at the upper third.

Olecranon. The point of the elbow bone.

Accessory carpal bone. The knee bones are composed of 2 rows: 4 bones in the upper row and 3 in the lower row. The accessory carpal bone is the outermost of the upper row.

Digit. The digit of the horse includes the long and short pastern bones and the coffin bone.

Bones of the hindlimb

The hindlimb is shown from the front and from the inside in Figs. 7 and 8, from the outside in Fig. 8, and from behind in Fig. 9.

Unlike the forelimb, the hindlimb is directly attached to the rest of the skeleton by a bone-to-bone joint, namely the thigh bone to the pelvis.

The pelvis is composed of three hip (coxal) bones, the sacrum and the three first tail bones (coccygeal vertebrae).

The paired coxal bones are the ilium, which forms the lateral wall, the ischium, which together with the pubis forms the floor of the pelvis. The roof is formed by the sacrum and the first three coccygeal vertebrae. The tuber coxae, the most lateral part of the pelvis, can be seen externally (Fig. 1).

The three coxal bones meet at the lower lateral corner of the pelvis to form the acetabulum. The acetabulum is the pelvic part of the hip joint.

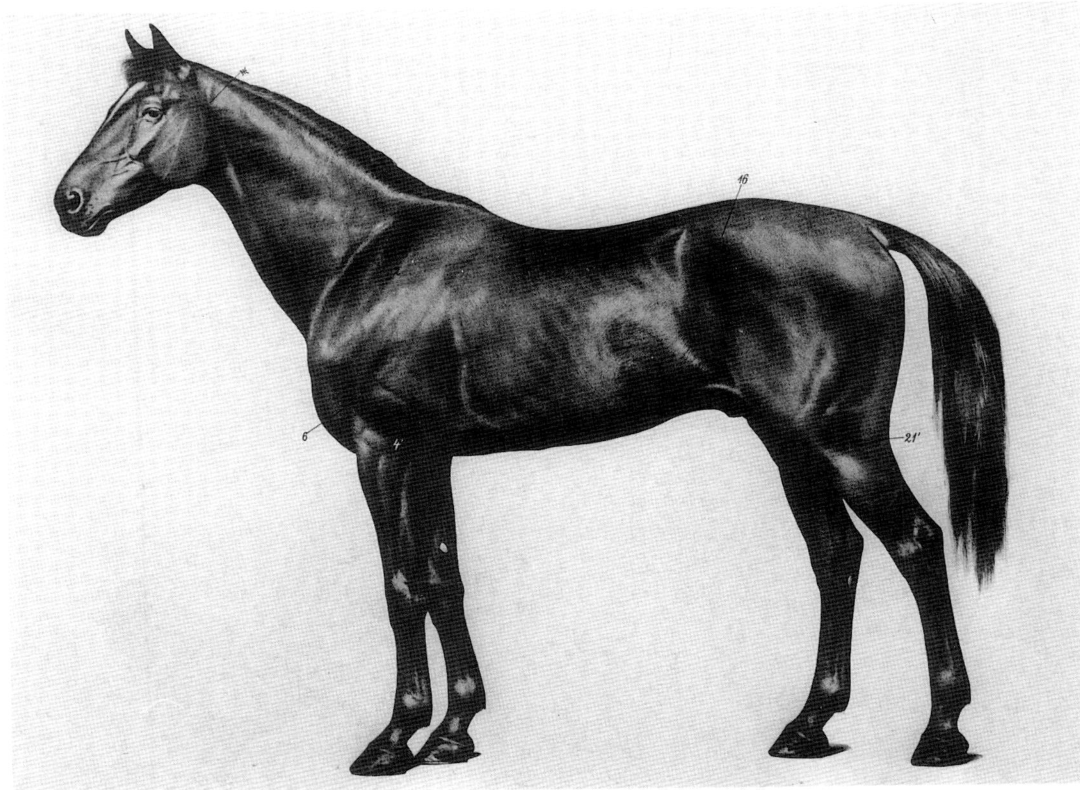

Fig. 1. Character at upper left points to the first cervical vertebra; 4′ Lateral epicondyle of humerus; 6 Deltoid tuberosity of humerus; 16 Tuber coxae; 21′ Lateral condyle of tibia.

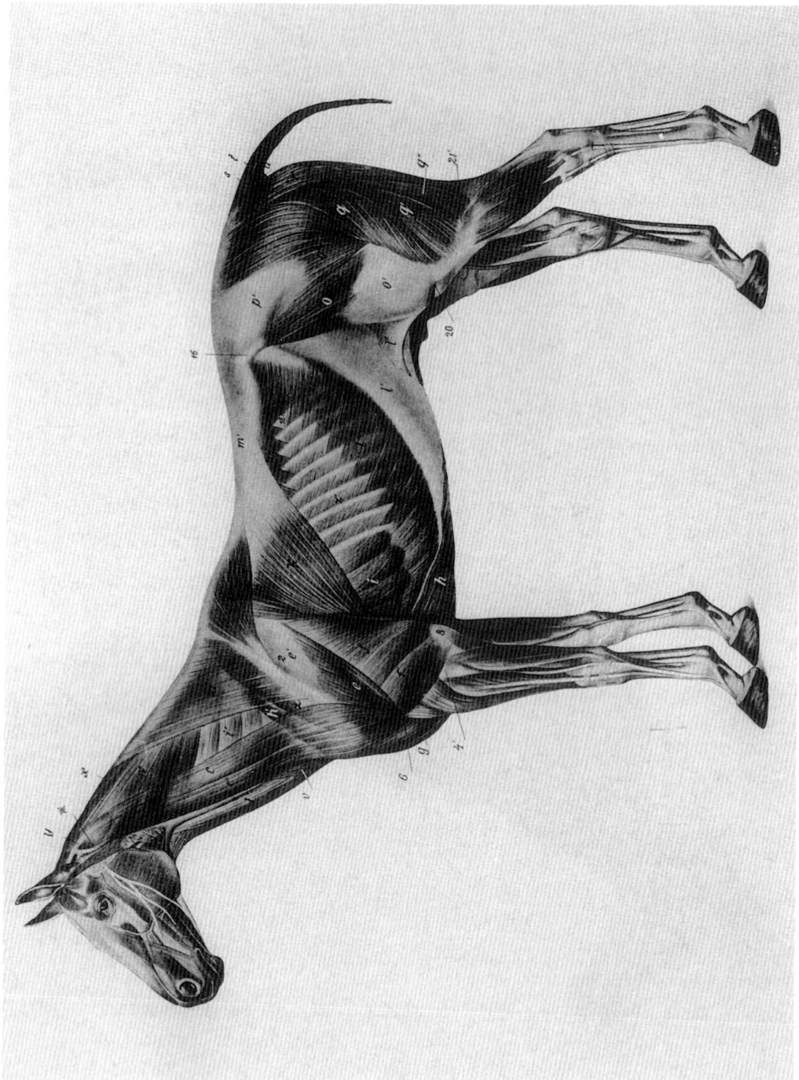

Fig. 2. Superficial dissection. Muscles. a Cervical part of trapezius; a′ Thoracic part of trapezius; c Omotransversarius; c′ Cleidomastoideus; d Sternocephalicus; 3, e′ Deltoideus; f Long head or triceps; f′ Lateral head of triceps; g Pectoralis descendens; h Pectoralis descendens; h′ Subclavius; i Thoracic part of serratus ventralis; i′ Cervical part of serratus ventralis; k Latissimus dorsi; l. External abdominal oblique; l′ Aponeurosis of external abdominal oblique; l″ Part of cutaneus trunci in fold of flank; m Serratus dorsalis; m′ Lumbodorsal fascia; o Tensor fasciae latae; o′ Fascia lata; o″ Gluteus superficialis; p′ Fascia over gluteus medius; q, q′, q″ Cranial, middle and caudal divisions of biceps femoris; r Semitendinosus; s Sacrocaudalis dorsalis lateralis; t Sacrocaudalis ventralis lateralis; u Coccygeus; v Cutaneus colli; w. Splenius; x Rhomboideus cervicis; y Tendon of longissimus capitis; z Supraspinatus.

Bones. 2 Spine of scapula; 4′ Lateral epicondyle of humerus; 6 Deltoid tuberosity; 8 Olecranon; 16 Tuber coxae; 20 Patella; 21′ Lateral condyle of tibia.

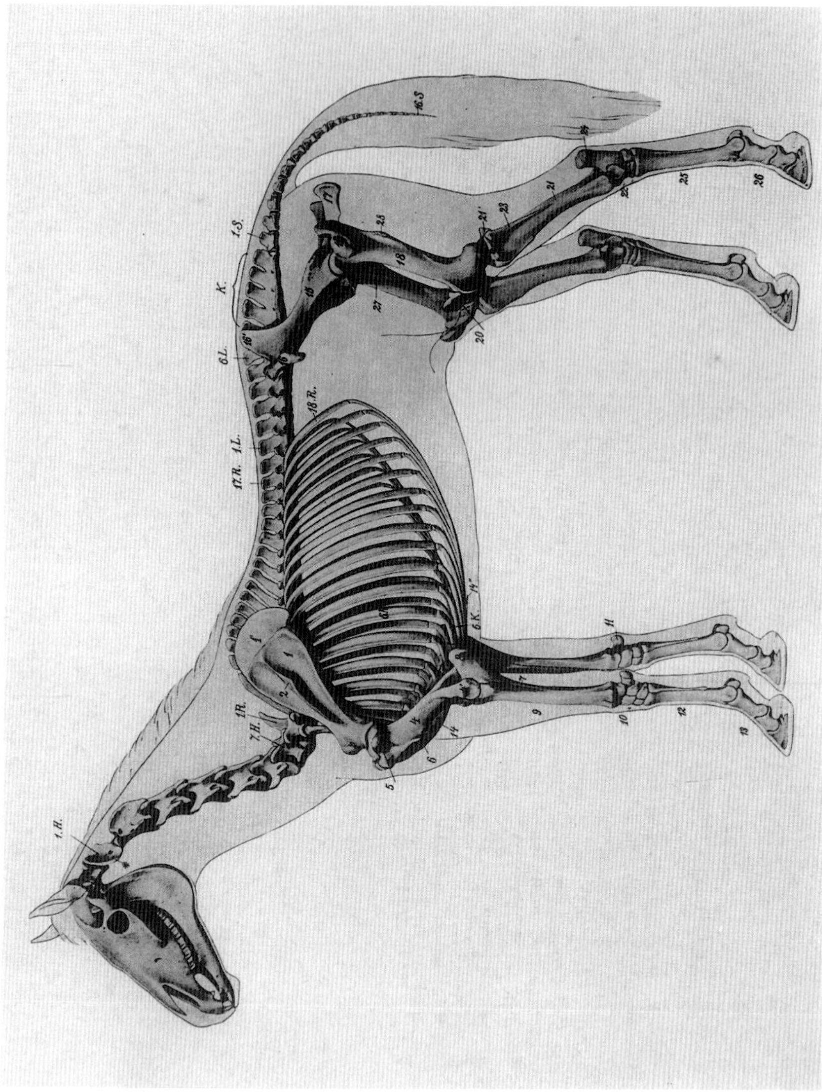
1.H.
7.H.
1R.
17.R.
1.L.
18.R.
6.L.
K.
1.S.
16.S
6.K.

Fig. 3. The skeleton of the horse seen from the left side. 1 Scapula; 1′ Scapular cartilage; 2 Spine of scapula; 4 Humerus; 4′ Lateral epicondyle of humerus; 5 Greater tubercle of humerus; 6 Deltoid tuberosity; 7 Ulna; 8 Olecranon; 9 Radius; 10 Carpus; 11 Accessory carpal bone; 12 Metacarpus; 13 Digit; 14 Sternum; 14″ Xiphoid cartilage; 15 Body of ilium; 16 Tuber coxae; 16′ Tuber sacrale; 17 Tuber ischiadicum; 18 Femur; 19 Greater trochaner of femur; 20 Patella; 21 Tibia; 21′ Lateral condyle of tibia; 22 Tarsus; 23 Fibula; 24 Tuber calcanei; 25 Metatarsus; 26 Digit; 27 Lesser trochanger of femus; 28 Trochanter tertius of femur; 1 H Atlas; 7 H. 7th cervical vertebra; K Sacrum; 6.K 6th costal cartilage; 1.L 1st lumbar vertebra; 6.L 6th lumbar vertebra; 1.R 1st thoracic vertebra; 6.R 6th rib; 18.R 18th rib; 1.S 1st coccygeal vertebra; 16.S 16th coccygeal vertebra; * Wing of atlas.

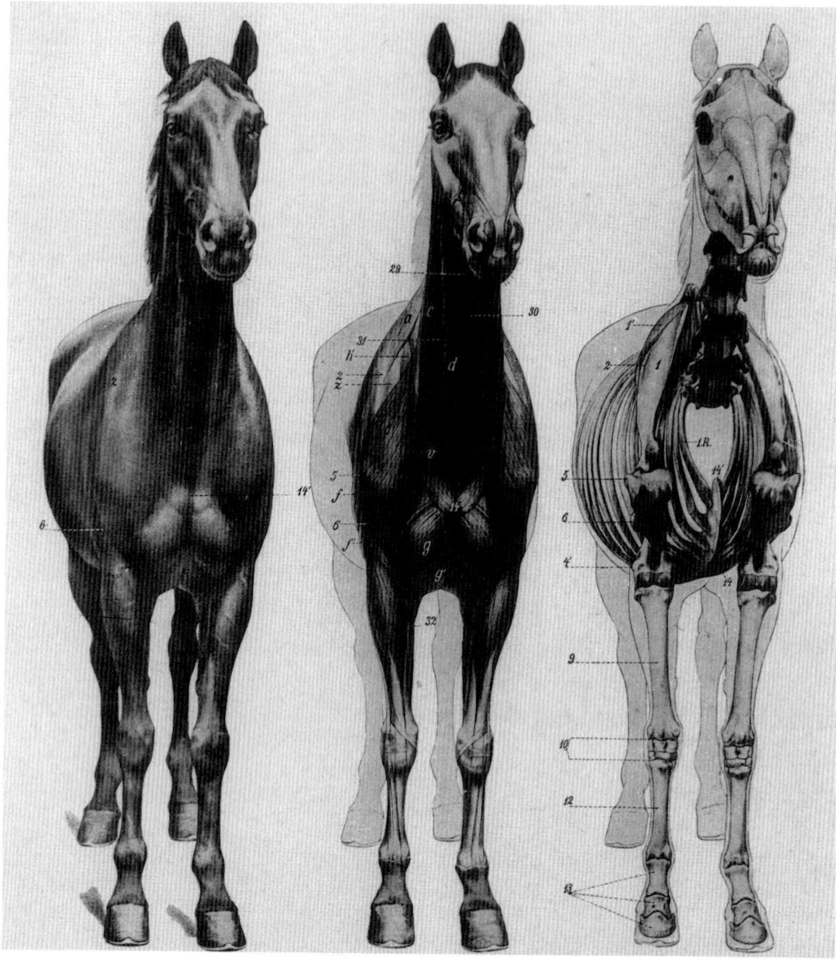

Fig. 4. Cranial view of the horse. Middle: Superficial dissection; Right: Skeleton.

Muscles. a Trapezius; c Cleidomastoideus; d Sternocephalicus; f Long head of triceps; f' Lateral head of triceps; g Pectoralis descendens; g' Pectoralis transversus; h' Subclavius; v Cutaneus colli; z Supraspinatus.

Bones. 1 Scapula; 1' Scapula cartilage; 2 Spine of scapula; 4 Humerus; 4' Lateral epicondyle of humerus; 5 Greater tubercle of humerus; 6 Deltoid tuberosity; 9 Radius; 10 Carpus; 12 Metacarpus; 13 Digit; 14 Sternum; 14' Manubrium sterni;

Other. 30 Sternohyoideus (muscle); 31 Jugular vein; 32 Cephalic vein. 1.R 1st rib.

The bones of the hindlimb are as follows:

Anatomical Name	*Popular Name*
Femur	Thighbone
Patella	Knee cap
Tibia	Leg bone
Fibula	Leg bone
Tarsus	Hock
Metatarsus III, MT III	Cannon bone
Metatarsus II and IV, MT II and MT IV	Splint bones
Proximal sesamoid bones	Sesamoid bones
1st phalanx, P I	Long pastern bone
2nd phalanx, P II	Short pastern bone
3rd phalanx, P III	Coffin bone
Distal sesamoid bone, navicular bone	Navicular bone

The knee cap, or patella, is by definition a sesamoid bone. The conventional use of "proximal sesamoid bones" for those at the lower end of the hindlimb cannon bones is, therefore, less than correct. The patella is more proximal. The tibia, or more correctly, the entire region between the stifle and the hock, is called the "gaskin" by horsemen.

Figs. 7-9 also name some, but far from all, anatomical details of the hind limb bones. Those named will be defined.

Lateral condyle of tibia. A projection or protrusion at the outside, upper end of the tibia.
Lateral malleolus of tibia. A rounded prominence on the outside of the lower end of the tibia.
Talus. Ankle.
Tuber calcanei. The point of the hock.
Tuber coxae. The most upwards and outwards point of the ilium.
Tuber sacrale. The most upwards and inwards point of the ilium.
Tuber ischiadicum. The lower, outwards point of the ischium.
Lateral condyle of femur. The outer, lower end of the femur which articulates with the tibia.
Greater trochanter of femur. A large process or protruberance on the outer, upper end of the thigh bone (femur).
Lesser trochanter of femur. A smaller process on the medial side below the neck of the femur.
Third trochanter; trochanter tertius of femur. A process on the outside of the thigh bone, just above the middle.

Joints

A joint is a place of union between two or more bones of the skeleton. The word articulation means exactly the same as joint.

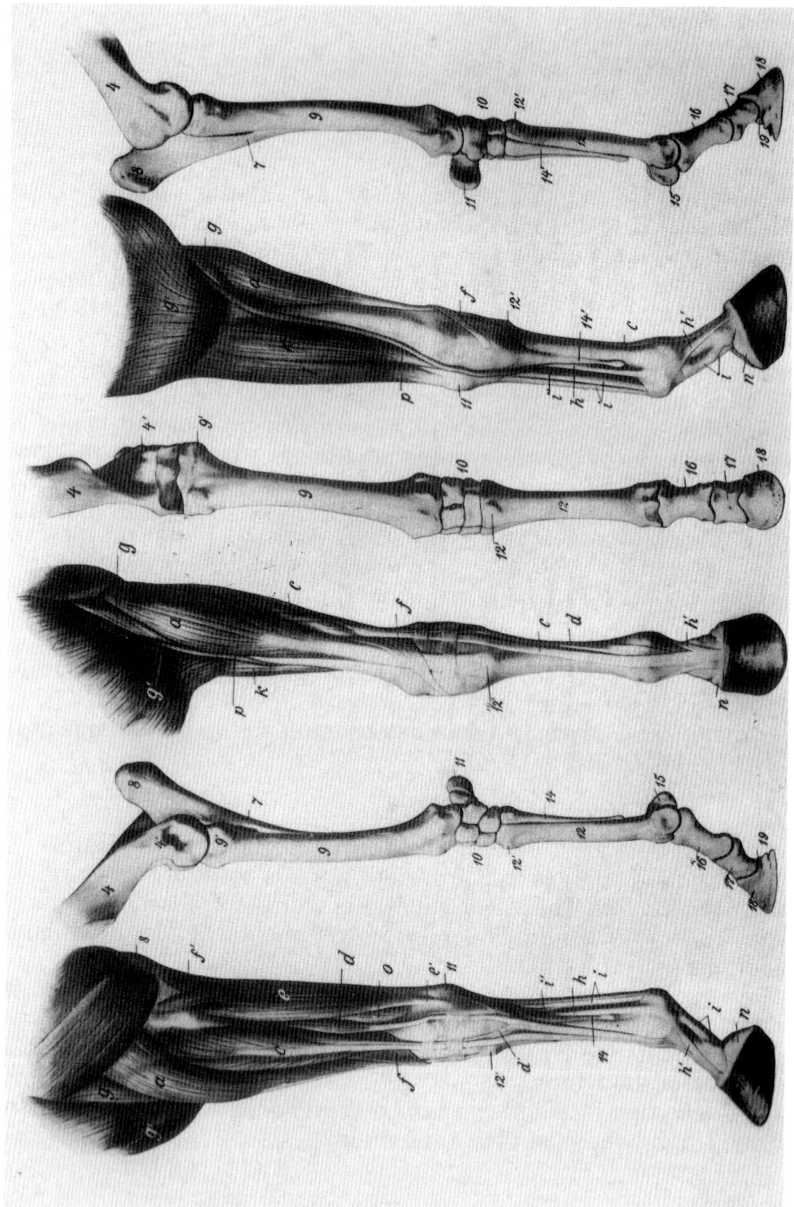

Fig. 5. Forelimb in lateral view (2 pictures to the left); in cranial view (2 pictures in center); and in medial view (2 pictures to the right).

Muscles. a Extensor carpi radialis; c Common digital extensor; d Lateral digital extensor; d′ Tendon of radial head of common digital extensor; 3, 3′ Ulnaris lateralis; f Extensor carpi obliquus; f′ Ulnar head of deep digital flexor; g Bracialis; g′ Pectoralis descendens and trasversus; h Interosseous; h′ Extensor branch of interosseous; i Superficial and deep flexor tendons; i′ Accessory ligament of deep flexor tendon; k Flexor carpi radialis; l Flexor carpi ulnaris; n Cartilage of hoof; o Deep digital flexor; p Cephalic vein.

Bones. 4 Humerus; 4′ Lateral epicondyle of humerus; 7 Ulna; 8 Olecranon; 9 Radius; 10 Carpus; 11 Accessory carpal bone; 12 MC III; 14 MC IV; 14′ Mc II; 15 Proximal sesamoid bones; 16 P I; 17 P II; 18 P III; 19 Navicular bone.

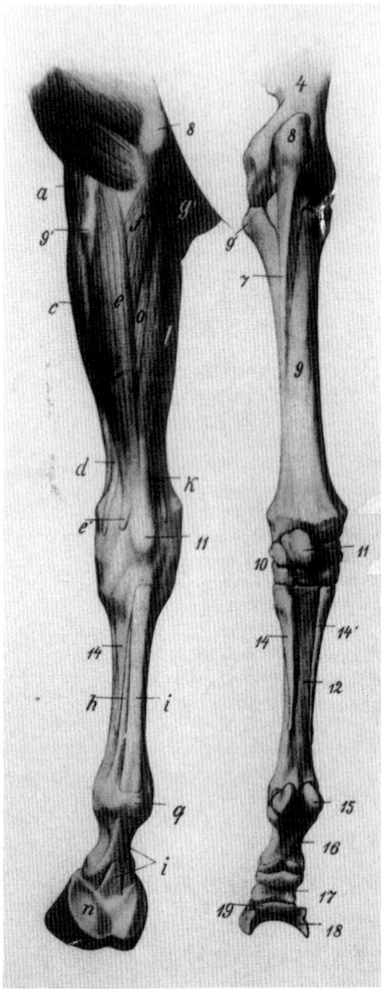

Fig. 6. Forelimb in caudal view. Muscles. a Extensor carpi radialis; c Common digital extensor; d Lateral digital extensor; e Ulnaris lateralis; f' Ulnar head of deep digital flexor; g Brachialis; g' Pectoralis descendens and transversus; h Interosseus; i Superficial and deep flexor tendons; k Flexor carpi radialis; 1 Flexor carpi ulnaris; n Cartilage of hoof; o Deep digital flexor; q Annular ligament of fetlock joint.

Bones. 4 Humerus; 7 Ulna; 8 Olecranon; 9 Radius; 9' Head of radius; 10 Carpus; 11 Accessory carpal bone; 12 MC III; 14 MC IV; 14' MC II; 15 Proximal sesamoid bones; 16 P I; 17 P II; 18 P III; 19 Navicular bone.

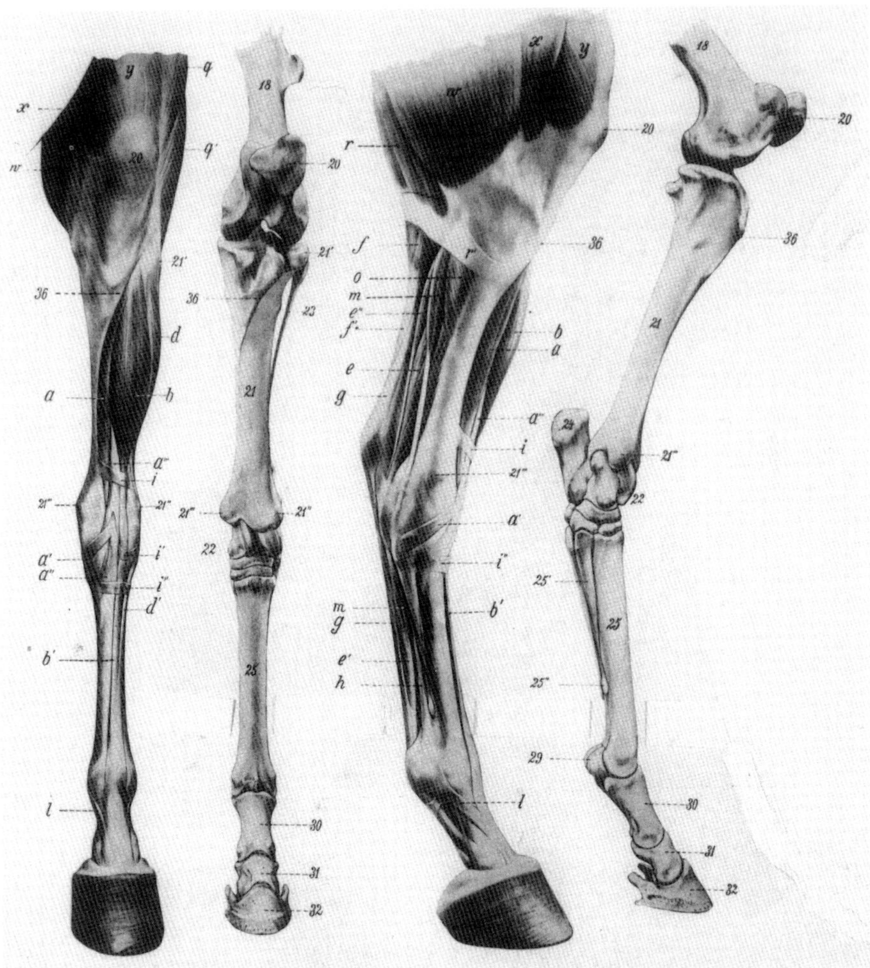

Fig. 7. Hindlimb in cranial view (2 pictures to the left) and in medial view (2 pictures to the right).

Muscles. a Tibialis cranialis; a′ Medial branch of tibialis cranialis tendon; a″ Dorsal branch of tibialis cranialis tendon; a″ ′ Peroneus tertius; b,b′ Long digital extensor; d,d′ Lateral digital extensor; e Deep head of deep digital flexor; e′ Deep digital flexor tendon; e″ Superficial head of deep digital flexor; f,f′ Medial head of gastrocnemius; g Superficial flexor tendon; h Interosseus; i,i′i″ Proximal, middle and distal retinacula; l Extensor branch of interosseus; m Medial head of deep digital flexor; o Popliteus; q,q′ Cranial and middle divisions of biceps femoris; r Semitendinosus; r′ Tibial tendon of semitendinosus; w Gracilis; x Sartorius; y Vastus medialis.

Bones. 18 Femur; 20 Patella; 21 Tibia; 21′ Lateral condyle of tibia; 21″ Lateral malleolus of tibia; 21″ ′ Medial malleolus of tibia; 22 Tarsus; 23 Fibula; 24 Tuber calcanei; MT III; 25′ MT II: 25″ Distal end of MT II; 29 Proximal sesamoid bones; 30 P I; 31 P II; 32 P III; 36 Tibial crest.

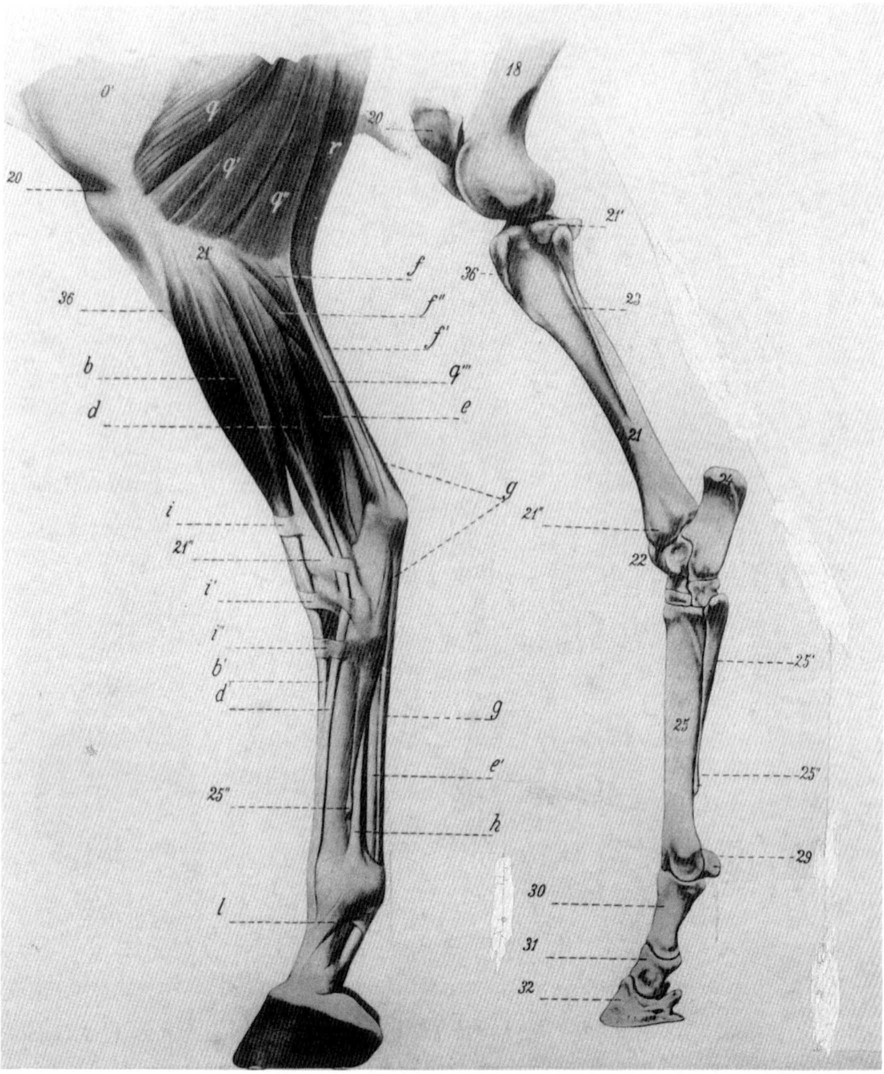

Fig. 8. Hindlimb in lateral view.

Muscles. b,b′ Long digital extensor; d,d′ Lateral digital extensor; e Deep head of deep digital flexor; e′ Deep digital flexor tendon; f,f′ Lateral head of gastrocnemius; f″ Soleus; g Superficial flexor tendon; h Interosseus; i,i′i″ Proximal, middle and distal retinacula; l Extensor branch of interosseus; o′ Fascia lata; q,q′,q″ Cranial, middle and caudal divisions of biceps femoris; l″ ′ Tarsal tendon of biceps femoris; r Semitendinosus.

Bones. 18 Femur; 20 Patella; 21 Tibia; 21′ Lateral condyle of tibia; 21″ Lateral malleolus of tibia; 22 Tarsus; 23 Fibula; 24 Tuber calcanei; 25 MT III; 25′ MT IV; 25″ Distal end of MT IV: 29 Proximal sesamoid bones; 30 PI; 31 P II; 32 P III; 36 Tibial crest.

A joint allows movements between bones in various directions. You will now be burdened with a few more terms.

Flexion. To bend; that is, to *decrease* the angle between bones or bend the leg.
Extension. To *increase* the angle between bones or to straighten the leg.
Rotation. Turning around an axis.
Abduction. Turning outwards.
Adduction. Turning inwards.
Circumdiction. The circular movement of a limb.

There are three types of joints in the limbs of the horse. They allow various movements of the joints.

A *ball and socket joint* is a joint in which the head of one bone plays (articulates) against the socket of another. The shoulder and hip joints are examples of this type of joint. A ball-and-socket joint allows movements in all directions.

A *hinge joint* allows movements only in one plane: flexion or extension.

A *gliding joint* is a joint between flat surfaces allowing only gliding movement.

Joints of the forelimb

The shoulder blade is attached to the body by muscles. There is no bone to bone joint. The joints are as follows:

Anatomical Name	*Popular Name*	*Type of joint*
Scapulo-humeral joint (scapula to humerus)	Shoulder joint	Ball-and-socket
Cubital joint (humerus to radius-ulna)	Elbow joint	Hinge
Radio-carpal (radius to upper row of carpal bones)	Knee joint	Hinge
Inter-carpal joint (upper to lower rows of carpal bones)	Knee joint	Hinge
Carpo-metacarpal joint (lower row of carpal bones to MC III)	Knee joint	Gliding
Metacarpo-phalangeal joint (MC III to P I)	Fetlock joint	Hinge
Proximal interphalangeal joint (P I to P II)	Pastern joint	Hinge
Distal interphalangeal joint (P II to P III)	Coffin joint	Hinge

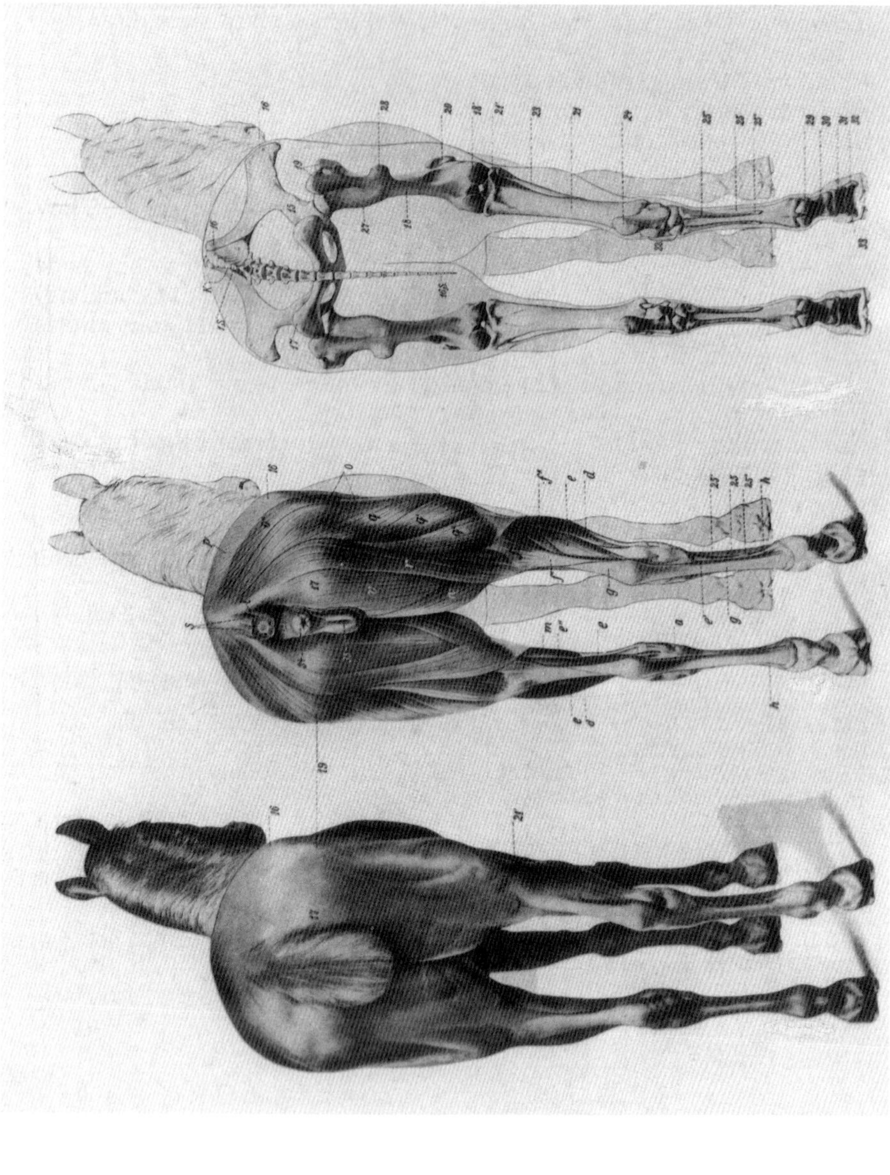

Fig. 9. Hindlimbs in caudal view.

Muscles. a Medial branch of tibialis cranialis tendon; d. Lateral digital extensor; e. Deep digital flexor; e′ Deep digital flexor tendon; e″ Tibialis caudalis; f Gastrocnemius; f′ Gastrocnemius tendon; f″ Soleus; g Superficial digital flexor tendon; h Interosseus; m Long digital flexor; o Tensor fasciae latae; o″ Gluteus superficialis; p′ Gluteus medius; q,q′,q″ Cranial, middle and caudal divisions of biceps femoris; r Semitendinousus; s,t Tail muscles; v Semimembranosus; w Gracilis.

Bones. 15 Body of ilium; 16 Tuber coxae; 16′ Tuber sacrale; 17 Tuber ischiadicum; 18 Femur; 18′ Lateral condyle of femur; 19 Greater trochanter of femur; 20 Patella; 21 Tibia; 21′ Lateral condyle of tibia; 22 Tarsus; 23 Fibula; 24 Tuber calcanei; 25 MT III; 25′ MT IV; 25″ Distal end of MT IV; 27 Lesser trochanter of femur; 28 Trochanter tertius of femur; 30 P I; 31 P II; 32 P III; K Sacrum; 1.S 1st coccygeal vertebra; 16.S 16th coccygeal vertebra.

Other. 34 Anus; 35 Vulva.

Joints of the hindlimb

Anatomical Name	*Popular Name*	*Type of joint*
Coxo-femoral joint (pelvis to femur)	Hip joint	Ball and socket
Genual joint (femur to patella; femur to tibia)	Stifle joint	Hinge and gliding
Tibio-tarsal joint (tibia to tarsus)	Hock	Hinge
Intertarsal joints (upper to lower rows of tarsal bones)	Hock	Hinge
Tarso-metatarsal joint (Tarsus to metatarsus)	Hock	Gliding
Metatarso-phalangeal joint (MT III to P I)	Fetlock joint	Hinge
Proximal interphalangeal joint (P I to P II)	Pastern joint	Hinge
Distal interphalangeal joint (P II to P III)	Coffin joint	Hinge

Muscles and tendons with action on the lower limb bones

Figs. 2 and 4-9 show, in addition to bones and joints, the muscles of the limbs. We will briefly describe only those involved in the motion of the lower limb bones, below the knee and hock. These are important in the future account of breakdowns.

The joints below the knee and the hock are all hinge joints that allow only extension and flexion.

The forelimb. There are two digital *extensor* muscles which straighten the leg, the common digital extensor and the lateral digital extensor. The common digital extensor (Figs. 5c and 6c) originates on the front aspect of the lower end of the arm bone, on the lateral part of the upper end of the forearm bone, and on the lateral part of the elbow bone (ulna). The muscular part ends near the lower end of the forearm bone, below which it continues as a tendon. At the knee, the tendon is outside but turns inwards to reach the midline near the fetlock joint. It continues downward to be attached to the upper end of the front aspect of all three digits, the long and short pastern bones and the coffin bone (Fig. 10). This muscle extends the digits and the knee and flexes the elbow.

The lateral digital extensor (Figs. 5d and 6d) originates on the lateral tuberosity of the lower end of the forearm bone, on the lateral border of the forearm bone, and on the shaft of the elbow bone. The lateral digital extensor muscle extends the digits and the knee. The muscular part terminates at the lower third of the forearm bone to become a tendon. The tendon of the lateral digital extensor joins that of the common digital extensor at the middle of the cannon bone (Fig. 7, d and d′).

There are two digital *flexor* muscles, a superficial and a deep. The superficial digital flexor originates on the medial epicondyle of the arm bone (the inner lowest part of the distal end) and the inner lower

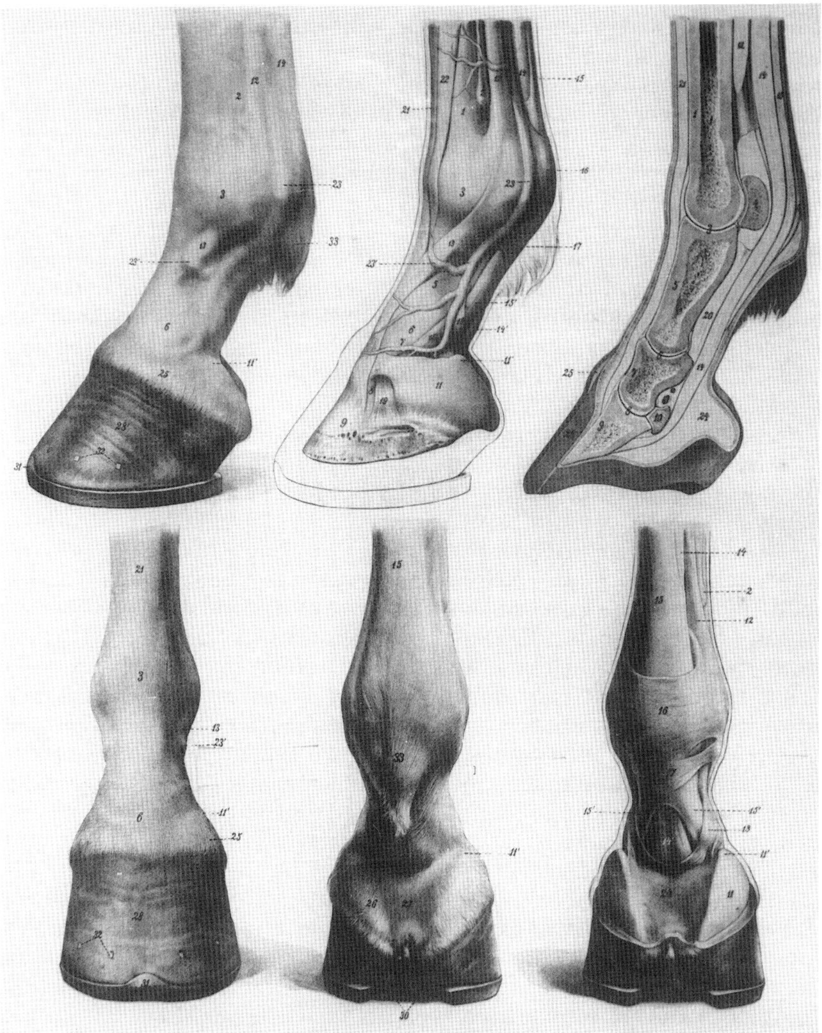

Fig. 10. Digit of the horse.

Upper row. Lateral view. Left: with skin, middle: superficial dissection; right: section slightly off mid-line.

Lower row. Left: cranial view; middle: caudal view; right: caudal view, superficial dissection.

1 MC III; 2 Distal end of MC IV; 3 Fetlock joint; 5 P I; 6 Pastern joint; 7 P II; 8 Coffin joint; 9 P III; 10 Navicular bone; 11,11′ Cartilage of hoof; 12 Interosseus; 13 Extensor branch of interosseus; 14,14′ Deep flexor tendon; 15,15′ Superficial flexor tendon; 16 Annular ligament of fetlock joint; 17 Proximal digital annular ligament; 18 Distal digital annular ligament; 19 Lateral collateral ligament of coffin joint; 20 Straight sesamoidean ligament; 21 Common digital extensor tendon; 22 Lateral digital extensor tendon; 23 Lateral digital vein; 23′ Dorsal branch to P I of lateral digital vein; 24 Digital cushion; 25 Coronet; 26 Bulb of heel; 27 Skin over digital cushion; 28 Toe; 28′ Lateral quarter; 28″ Medial heel; 20 Sole, actually apex of frog; 30 Base of frog; 31 Chip of shoe; 32 Clinches of nails; 33 Ergot, surrounded by the fetlock; 34 Depression distal to the distal end of MC IV or II.

part of the forearm bone. As it approaches the knee, it narrows into a tendon (Figs. 5i and 6i). The tendon runs on the back side of the cannon bone as the most superficial tendon just beneath the skin. The tendon attaches to the lower back side of the long pastern bone and to the upper part of the back side of the short pastern bone (Fig. 10). The action of the superficial digital flexor is to bend the digits and to straighten the elbow.

The deep digital flexor (Figs. 5f′, 6f′, 5o and 6o) bends the foot and the knee and straightens the elbow. It also originates on the medial epicondyle of the arm bone, on the inner part of the upper end of the elbow bone (olecranon), and on the middle of the back side of the forearm bone. The muscular part ends about 4 inches above the knee and the deep digital flexor continues downward as a tendon. The tendon (Figs. 5c and 6c) runs inside the superficial digital flexor, goes through a ring formed by the superficial digital flexor tendon, and attaches to the back side of the coffin bone (Fig. 10). As stated above, the deep digital flexor flexes the digits and the knee and extends the elbow.

The suspensory ligament supports the fetlock joint and prevents too much flexion or extension. The suspensory ligament is a highly modified muscle. Few muscle fibers remain and the structure is usually referred to as a ligament. It originates on the lower half of the back side of the lower row of knee bones and on the upper back end of the cannon bone. It runs downward as a thick band inside the deep flexor tendon and, about ¾ down on the cannon bone, divides into two branches. Each branch embraces the upper and outer and inner corner of the respective sesamoid bone and then continues downward and forward to join the extensor tendon on the front end of the long pastern bone (Figs. 5h, h′, 6h, h′, Fig. 10). These branches are also referred to as the extensor branches of the suspensory ligament (Fig. 5, h′).

The hindlimb. There are two digital *extensor* or straightening muscles: the long digital extensor and the lateral digital extensor. The long digital extensor (Figs. 7b, b′ and 8b, b′) originates at the lower front end of the thigh bone between the lateral epicondyle and the trochlea of the femur; the area is called the extensor fossa. The belly of the muscle narrows into a tendon just above the hock. The tendon runs downward over the front of the hock. It is attached to the top front end of all three digital bones: the long and short pastern bones and the coffin bone. It extends (straightens) the digit and flexes (bends) the hock.

The lateral digital extensor (Figs. 7d, d′, 8d, d′ and 9d) originates on the lateral ligament of the stifle, on the fibula, on the lateral border of the tibia, and on the suspensory ligament. The belly ends at the lower quarter of the tibia. The tendon, present in the entire muscular part, runs downward on the outer part of the hock, turns inward and joins the tendon of the long digital extensor above the middle of the cannon bone. It also acts to straighten the foot and bend the hock.

There are two digital *flexor* muscles which bend the foot and straighten the hock. They are the superficial digital flexor and the deep digital flexor. The superficial digital flexor (Figs. 7g, 8g and 9g) originates in the supracondylar fossa of the thigh bone, a ditch on the back side of the thigh bone just above the lateral condyle. The muscular belly is poorly developed and is mostly tendon. It is attached to the point of the hock and then runs downward to end like its forelimb counterpart.

The deep digital flexor (Figs. 7c, c′, c″, m, 8c′, 9c, c′c″,m) originates on the back side of the lateral condyle of the tibia, on the middle third of the back surface of the tibia, on the upper lateral border of the tibia, on the back border of the fibula, and on the suspensory ligament. The muscular parts end at the lower third of the tibia, and the continuing tendon is attached like its forelimb counterpart. The action of the deep digital flexor is to flex the digit and to extend the hock.

The suspensory ligament (Figs. 7h, 1, 8h, 1) originates on the lower half of the back side of the 3rd tarsal bone (the largest bone of the lower row of hock bones) and on the uppermost part of the back side of the cannon bone. From here downward, its course and attachments are the same as those of the forelimb. Again, the suspensory ligament supports the fetlock joint.

REFERENCES

1. Ellenberger, W., H. Baum and H. Dittrich. 1949. An Atlas of Animal Anatomy for Artists. Second edition. Dover Publications, Inc. NY.
2. Sisson and Grossman's The Anatomy of the Domestic Animals. 1975. 5th edition. Getty, R., ed. W.B. Saunders Co., Philadelphia, London and Toronto.

The above references are also used in forthcoming chapters but will not be repeated.

III. DEVELOPMENT OF BONES

1. Introduction

Bones are organs which consist of the tissue bone, cartilage, bone marrow, nerves, blood vessels, and the surrounding bone membrane, the periosteum. Cartilage is defined as a translucent elastic tissue that composes most of the skeleton of the embryo, and becomes for the most part converted into bone in higher vertebrates.

There are two types of development of bones: within membranes and within cartilage; the latter is called endochondral development of bones. ALL LIMB BONES DEVELOP WITHIN CARTILAGE.

2. Types of bones

The limb bones are classified according to shape:

Long bones: bones in which the length is markedly greater than the width. The long bones are the arm bone, forearm bones, the thigh bone, the tibia, the cannon bone, and the long and short pastern bones.

Short bones: bones with the three dimensions about equal. The short bones are the bones of the knee, the hock, and the coffin bone.

Flat bones: bones more or less in the shape of a plate. There is one flat bone of each forelimb, the shoulder blade.

Sesamoid bones: bones within tendons.

3. Development of long bones

a. Development of the shaft

i. *The cartilage model.* Cartilage develops early in the limb buds of the embryo. The fertilized egg is called an embryo during the first weeks of pregnancy. From here on to foaling, it is called a fetus. In the early stage, the cartilage cells are small and arranged haphazardly. The cartilage appears as a dark area without any specific features in the low-power microscopic field. This is illustrated in Fig. 11, which shows the forelimb of an 85-day-old thoroughbred fetus of about 4 and 5⁄16 inches crown-to-rump length. The section is from front to back and slightly off the midline. From the bottom of the picture, you see the coffin bone, the short and long pastern bones (the sesamoid bones are not in the section), the cannon bone, the knee bones, and the

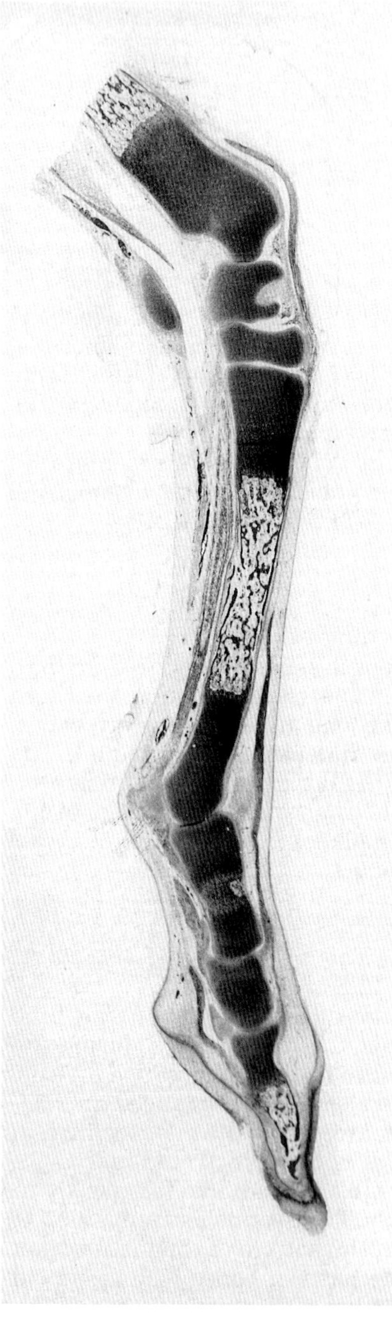

Fig. 11. Lengthwise section of the forelimb of an 85-day-old thoroughbred fetus; cranial is to the right, palmar is to the left. From bottom are the coffin bone, the short pastern, and the long pastern bones. Then the cannon bone, the knee bones, and the lower part of the forearm bone appear. The dark areas are cartilage. In the coffin bone, ossification has begun in the lower ⅔, has not yet begun in the short pastern bone, and is just beginning in the long pastern bone—see the light area in the middle of the bone. In the cannon bone, ossification is well advanced in the middle. The knee bones have not yet started to ossify. The forearm bone is well under way to convert into bone.

The section is a microscopic preparation cut at about two-thousandths of an inch and stained with hematoxylin and eosin. The microscopic picture was then reproduced at a magnification of 8 times. In future microscopic pictures, only the magnification will be given. If another stain is used, it will be identified.

lower end of the forearm bone. The cartilage model, shown as the dark area, is surrounded by a thin membrane, the perichondrium. The perichondrium is not visible in Fig. 11.

ii. *The bone collar.* The first sign of conversion of cartilage into bone (ossification) appears on the cranial surface of the mid-portion of the cartilage model, which, at that time, is roughly cylindrical. The cells of the perichondrium assume the role of osteoblasts and lay down a layer of bone (Fig. 12). This bone is called the bone collar and is

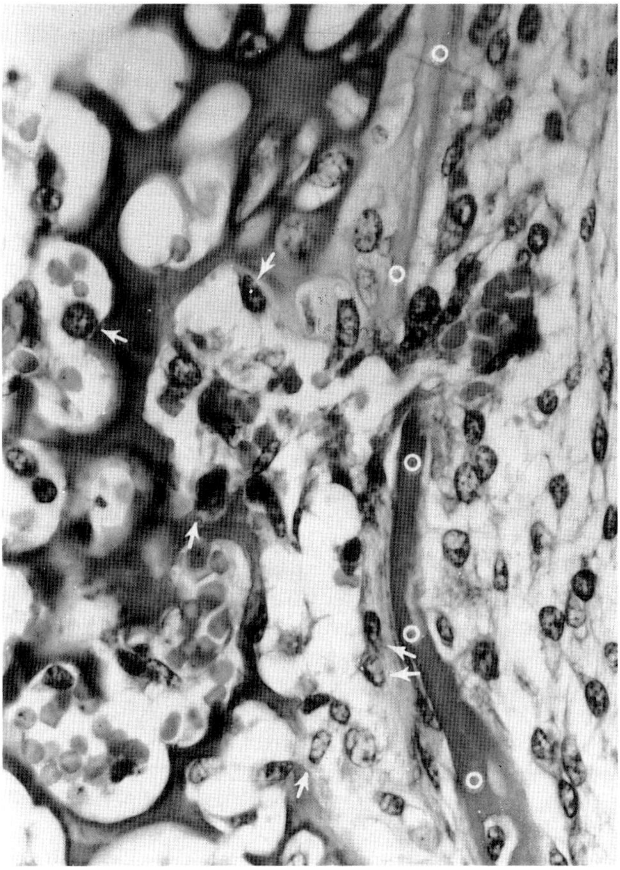

Fig. 12. Same specimen as in Fig. 11, at the front end of the long pastern bone. The bone collar is indicated by circles. At about the middle of the section to the right is a gap in the bone collar; this is destined to become the nutrient foramen. The cartilage cells are dead, but the core between these cells remains. Osteoblasts (indicated by arrows) lay down bone on these cores. ×640.

destined to become the shaft of a long bone. The bone collar is formed early in embryonic life, and its appearance varies greatly among the bones. Seen in Fig. 11 as a light area it is barely beginning to appear in the long pastern bone of an 85-day-old fetus, is advanced in the cannon and forearm bones, but has not yet appeared in the short pastern bone.

Once bone has been formed by the perichondrium, its name is changed to periosteum. In Fig. 12, there is a gap in the bone collar through which blood vessels enter into and exit from the cartilage model. This gap is called the nutrient foramen.

As the bone collar is formed, the cartilage cells next to the collar undergo a sequence of changes. The cells swell and eventually die. The death of a cell is seen in the microscopic slide by loss of the nucleus. The core between the cells becomes calcified, and though cartilage cells break up, the calcified core remains. The space of the dead cartilage cells is then invaded by blood vessels coming in through the nutrient foramen. Fetal bone marrow accompanying the blood vessels fills the spaces left behind the dead cartilage cells. Osteoblasts are bone forming cells. They are components of this incoming tissue which locate on the cartilage core and begin to lay down bone matrix. The events are shown in Fig. 12.

iii. *The ossification center.* Following the formation of the bone collar and the ossification of nearby cells, on the outside of the model, an ossification center appears in the middle at the midpoint of the cylindrical cartilage model. The ossification is preceded by continuous changes in the cartilage that is well away from the center.

The length of the cannon bone in the 85-day-old fetus in Fig. 11 is 3/8 of an inch (the picture is enlarged 8 times). During the next 250 days, this cannon bone will grow to 11 inches, the average length of that bone of a thoroughbred horse at birth, an increase in length by 30 times. This growth, obviously, requires a great rate of increase in the number of cartilage cells. The process is shown in Fig. 13. The cartilage cells are relatively small, and the core between the cells is relatively abundant. Cartilage cells increase in number by cell division, or mitosis. Closer to the ossification center, the cartilage cells swell and arrange in columns (Fig. 14). The core becomes relatively less abundant but does persist between the columns. As the columns approach the ossification center, swelling and ballooning of the cartilage cells become more prominent (Fig. 15). These disintegrating cells break up, and the spaces formed by the break-ups are filled with bone marrow. The cartilage cores between the cells continue as straight projections into the marrow space. Osteoblasts lay down bone matrix on these cores, and bars of bone are formed. The ossification proceeds upward and downward, and the bone increases in length. As this happens, the formation of the bone collar extends upward and downward and is always one step ahead of the advancing bars of bone (Fig. 16). These

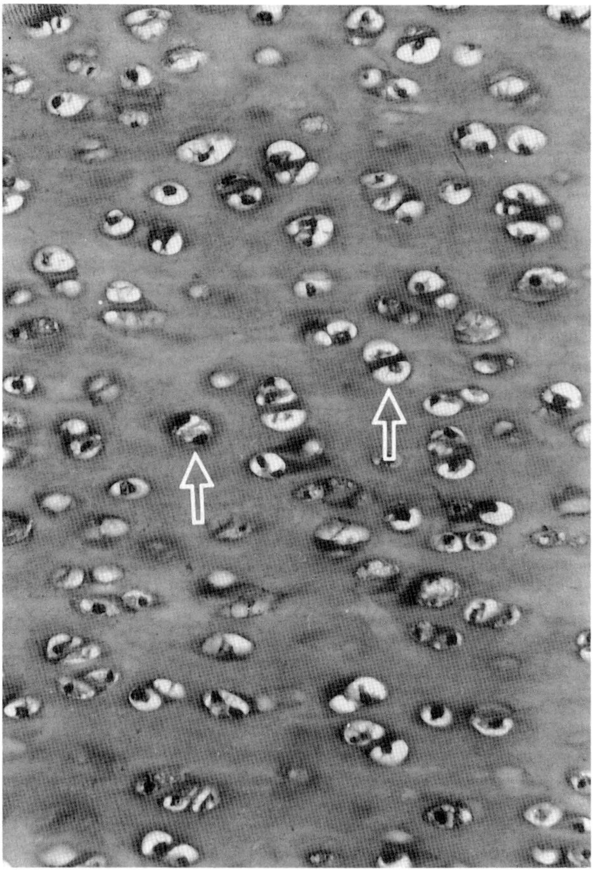

Fig. 13. Same specimen as in Fig. 11. We are now looking at the cartilage away from the ossification front. The cartilage cells are dividing at a very high rate. In front of arrows are cells in late stage of division. ×300.

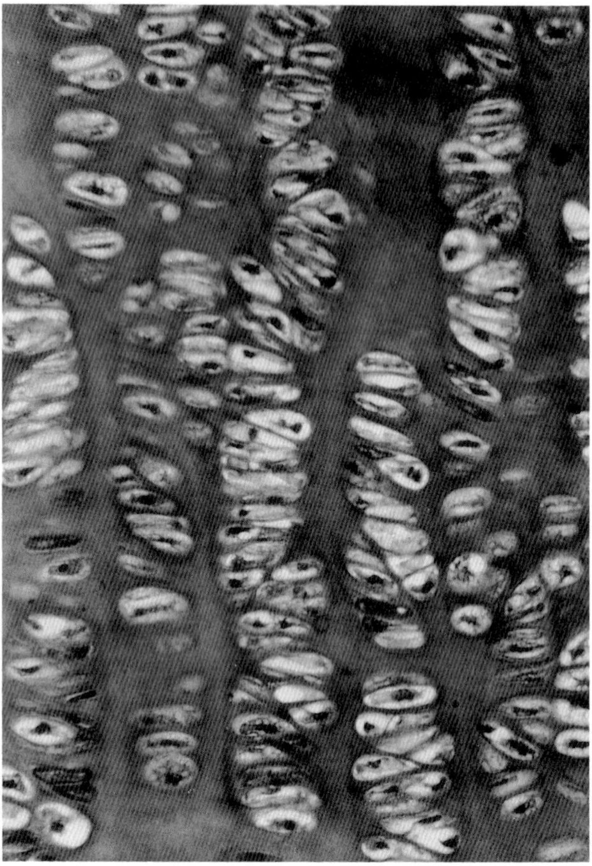

Fig. 14. Same specimen as in Fig. 11. This area is closer to the ossification front. The cartilage cells enlarge and arrange themselves in columns. ×300.

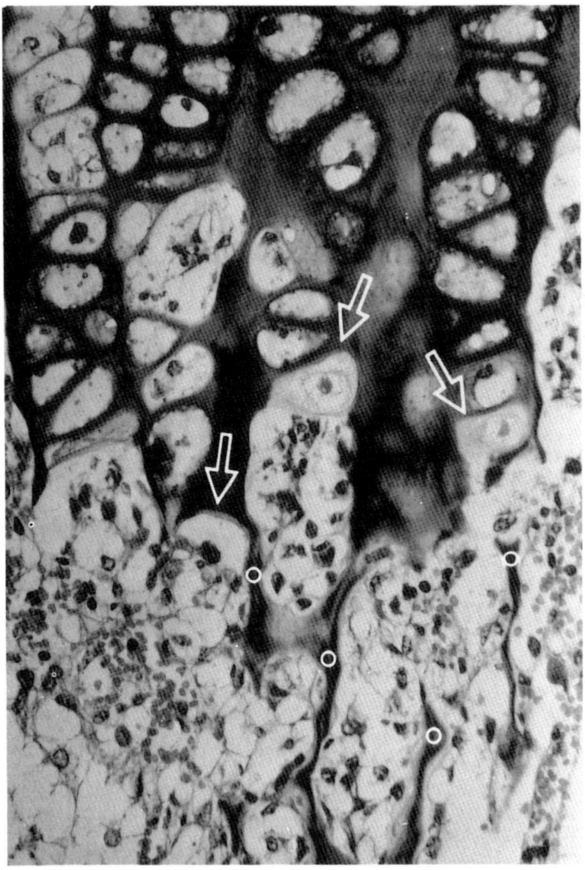

Fig. 15. Same section as in Fig. 11. We are now looking at the area where cartilage cells start to produce bone. The cartilage cells at top are enlarged and are dying. The cells in front of arrows are penetrated by blood vessels. The cartilage core, indicated by circles, descends. Osteoblasts lay down bone on these cores. ×300.

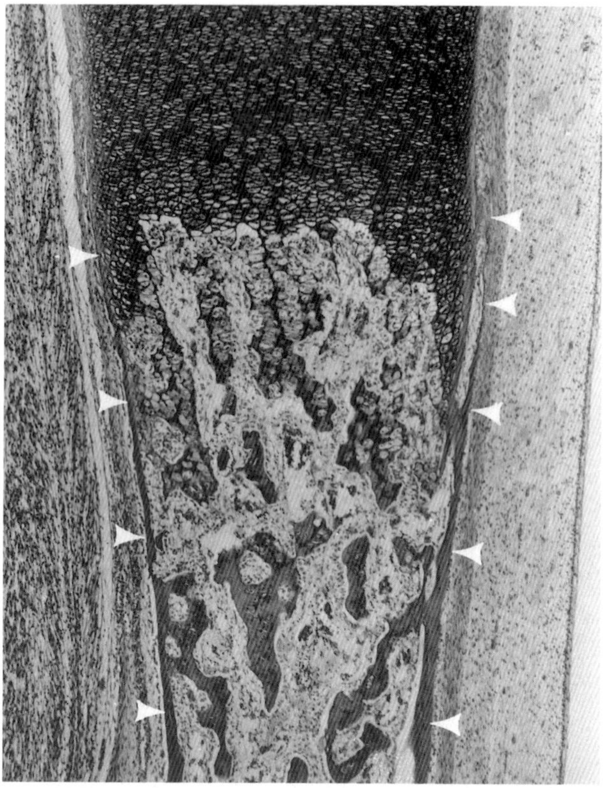

Fig. 16. Same section as in Fig. 11. The dark area at the top is cartilage. The thin band in front of the arrows is the bone collar. Note that the formation of the bone collar is one step ahead of the conversion of cartilage into bone. ×45.

trabeculae are removed or resorbed as they achieve a certain length and the marrow space is thus formed.

The upward and downward expansion of the ossification is limited by the events in the ends of the cartilage model. Ossification centers appear in the ends of long bones in the cartilage model considerably later than in the middle. In the arm bone, the forearm bone, the thigh bone, and the tibia, ossification centers appear in both ends. In the cannon bone, an ossification center appears only in the lower end, and in the long and short pastern bones only in the upper end.

The ossification process in the ends of long bones is similar to that described for the middle part of the cartilage model. In the lower end of the cannon bone of a 283-day-old fetus, the ossification center is well established (Fig. 17) but the final shape is not yet suggested. At birth, some 50 days later, the radiographic picture defines the final

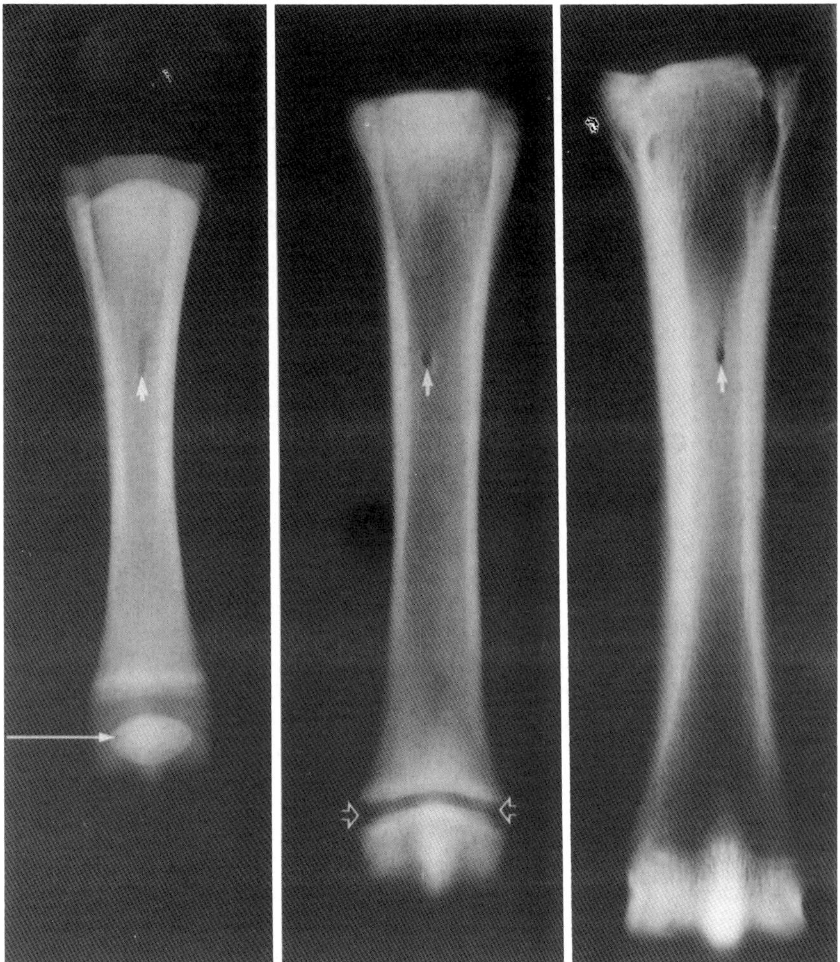

Fig. 17. This picture shows radiographs of the cannon bone of a front leg of a 283-day-old fetus (left), of a 1-day-old colt (middle), and of a 2-year-old filly (right).

The nutrient foramen (short arrows) is placed at the same horizontal level in the figures. In the fetus, the ossification center (long arrow) is well established, but its final shape has not yet been achieved. At birth (middle part) the ossification center at the lower end is almost complete. Note that the age difference between the cannon bones in the radiographs to the left and in the middle is only 7 weeks. At birth, the growth plate between the open arrows appears as a negative image in the radiograph. In the mature cannon bone (right), the growth plate is closed.

There is a growth plate only at the lower end of the cannon bone—this is the reason for the upward "migration" of the nutrient foramen. Note also that little lengthwise growth of the cannon bone takes place between birth and maturity.

shape of the lower part of the cannon bone. Note that there is cartilage between the two approaching ossification centers. Some 7 months later, the cannon bone has achieved its adult shape. The radiographic picture of the cannon bone in a 2-year-old filly is shown in Fig. 17. In the mature bone, no cartilage separates the lower end from the rest of the bone. Note that the growth in length of the cannon bone from birth to maturity is minimal, no more than one inch.

Microscopic examination reveals what happened during this maturation process. Fig. 18 shows the lower part of the cannon bone in a 283-day-old fetus. The circles indicate the border between the ossification centers from the shaft downward and from the lower end. Tiny bone bars are formed toward the shaft (upward), and they become thicker with increasing distance from the cartilage. The cartilage of the lower end, the black area below the circles, is still present, but irregularly arranged trabeculae are also present. The cartilage of the upper part, that is the cartilage derived from the middle of the cylinder, is now called a growth plate.

iv. *The growth plate.* Whereas the cartilage model has been ossified at a great speed, the growth persists for a long time. The zone away from the ossification center (lower part in Fig. 19) is where cell division occurs and where growth in length is initiated. The cells then become larger and arrange in distinct columns (Fig. 19, middle part) and then, finally, become blistered (vesiculated). At the ossification zone the cells die and the core between the cartilage cells becomes calcified. Cartilage cores project from the growth plate, and osteoblasts lay down bone on these cores. Note that the trabeculae formed in this way are arranged perpendicularly to the growth plate (Fig. 19).

When growth ceases, an event caused by hormones, the growth plate gradually becomes narrower and, finally, disappears. This is called closure of the growth plate, after which growth in length can no longer occur. After this closure, bone trabeculae from both ossification centers meet to form one unit (Fig. 20).

As mentioned above, the growth plate of the cannon bone closes at about 7 months of age. In the other long bones of the limbs, closure occurs later. In the arm bone, the upper growth plate closes at about 3½ years and the lower one at about 1½ years of age. In the main forearm bone, the radius, the upper growth plate closes before the lower one. Thus, the arm bone and the forearm bone grow toward the elbow. The nutrient foramen is, consequently, located below the midpoint of the armbone and above the midpoint of the forearm bone. In the hind limbs, the closure of the growth plate of the upper end of the thigh bone occurs earlier than in the lower end. In the tibia, the upper growth plate closes earlier than the lower one. This means that the thigh bone and the tibia grow away from the stifle. The difference in time of closure of the upper and lower growth plates is, however, much

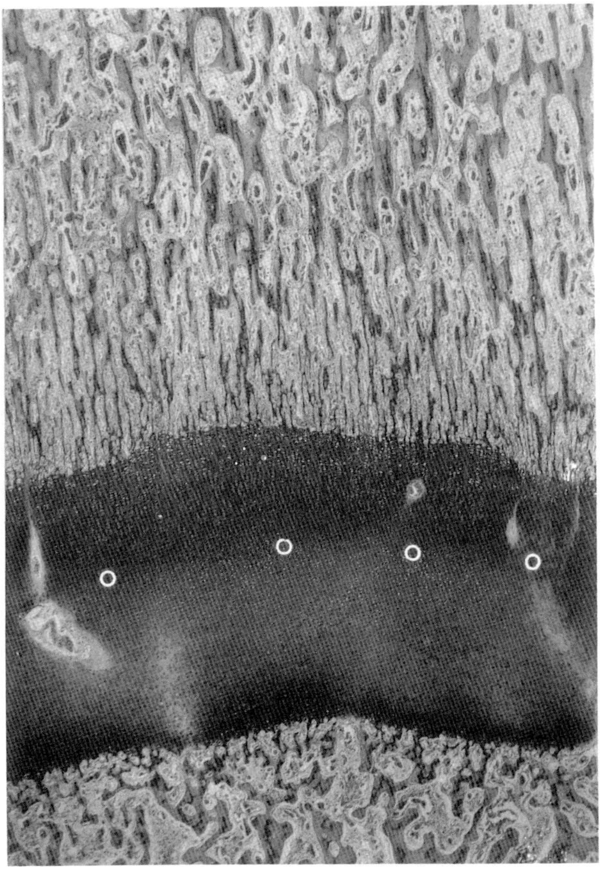

Fig. 18. The lower part of the cannon bone of a 1-day-old thoroughbred colt. The circles indicate the border between the cartilage of the shaft (black area above the circles) and the cartilage from the lower end (below the circles). The cartilage is producing bone bars projecting into the shaft (upward). The lower part depicts bone formation of the lower end of the cannon bone. ×10.

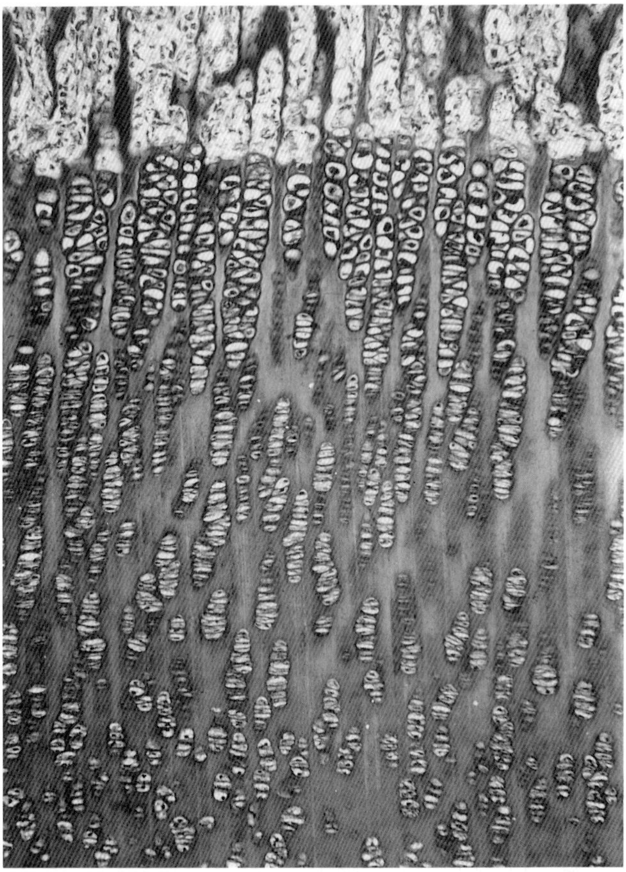

Fig. 19. Same specimen as in Fig. 18, cartilage facing the shaft, but at higher magnification. The cartilage is now called a growth plate. Cells at the bottom proliferate, line up in columns, become vesiculated, and die; trabeculae are formed on the continuing bars of cartilage core. ×110.

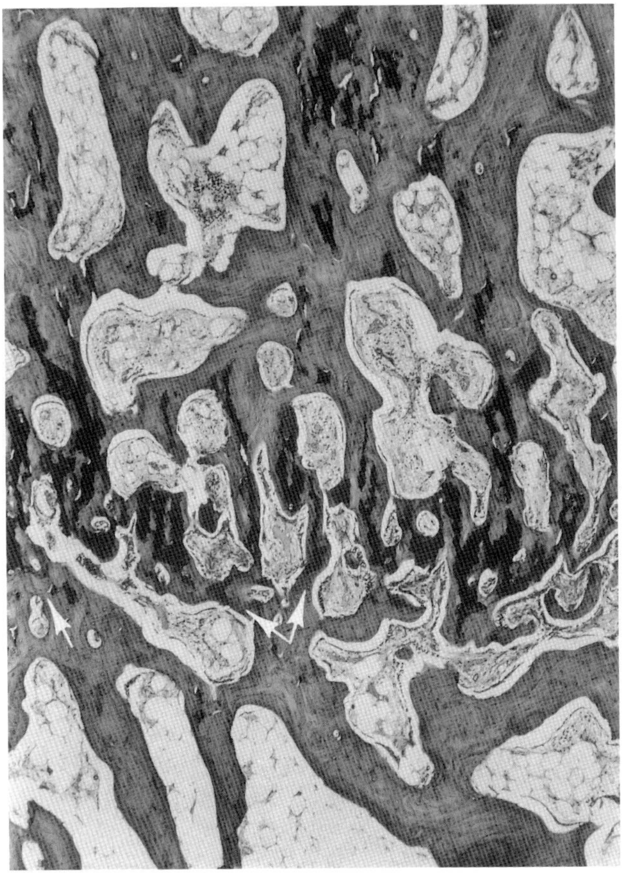

Fig. 20. Lower part of cannon bone in a 7-month-old pony colt. The growth plate is closed. The arrow points to bony bars with black material in the center, which is retained cartilage. This indicated the previous site of the growth plate. The bony bars now form one unit. ×40.

less than that in the corresponding bones of the front leg. Consequently, the nutrient foramen in the thigh bone and in the tibia are much closer to the midpoint than in the arm bone and the forearm bone.

Now back to the ossification center in the end of long bones. In the 283-day-old fetus, ossification is advanced but a thick layer of cartilage still exists facing the shaft (Fig. 18) and facing the joint (Fig. 21). In Fig. 21, the bony bars are slender with haphazard orientation. At birth, the extension of the ossification has almost reached its final stage (Fig. 22). The trabeculae are much thicker, and they are arranged perpendicularly to the cartilage. The remaining cartilage is destined to become the joint cartilage.

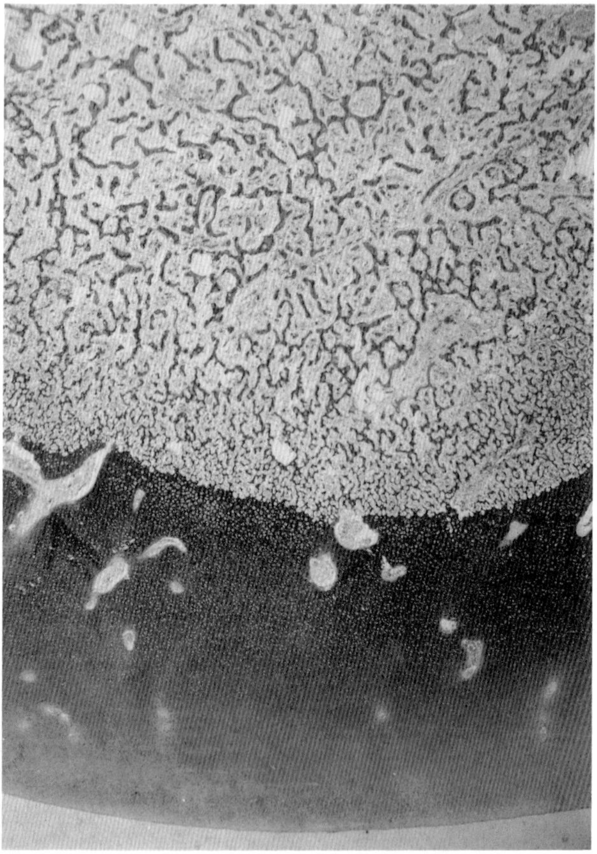

Fig. 21. Lowest part of the cannon bone of a 283-day-old thoroughbred fetus. The cartilage (black area at bottom) is thick, and the bony bars above are slender. ×10.

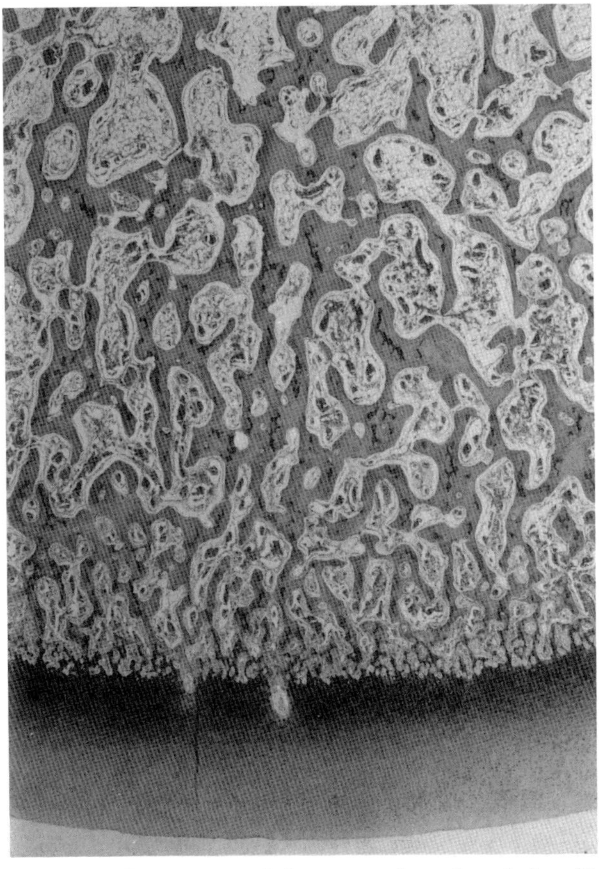

Fig. 22. Lowest part of the cannon bone in a 1-day-old thoroughbred colt. The cartilage at the bottom is relatively thin, and the bony bars are thicker and generally arranged perpendicularly to the cartilage. ×16.

The joint cartilage and adjacent structures in the mature horse are shown in Fig. 23. The inner part of the cartilage is calcified, and is called the zone of calcified cartilage. Just beneath that structure is a thick subchondral bone plate. This unit, (the joint cartilage, the zone of calcified cartilage, and the subchondral bone plate), is supported by trabeculae arranged perpendicularly (Fig. 24).

The growth activity in the ossification center in the end of a long bone contributes only little, about 3 percent, to the total growth in length of a long bone.

If there is no ossification center in one end of a long bone, the ossification process from the shaft continues, and that cartilage will eventually form the joint cartilage.

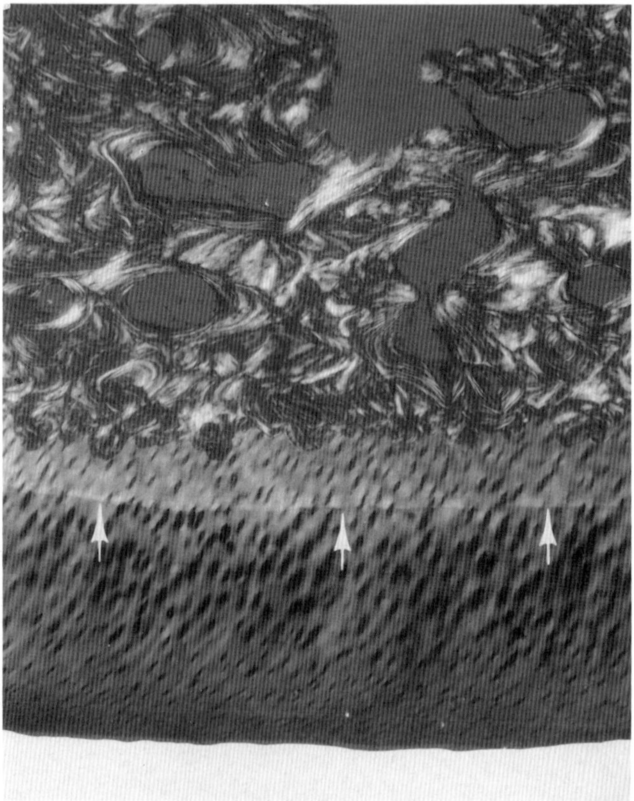

Fig. 23. Lowest part of the cannon bone in a 3-year-old thoroughbred gelding. The cartilage is at bottom. The arrows indicate the sharp demarcation between the joint cartilage (below) and the zone of calcified cartilage. Tightly adhered to that zone is the subchondral bone plate. ×45, specimen exposed with polarized light.

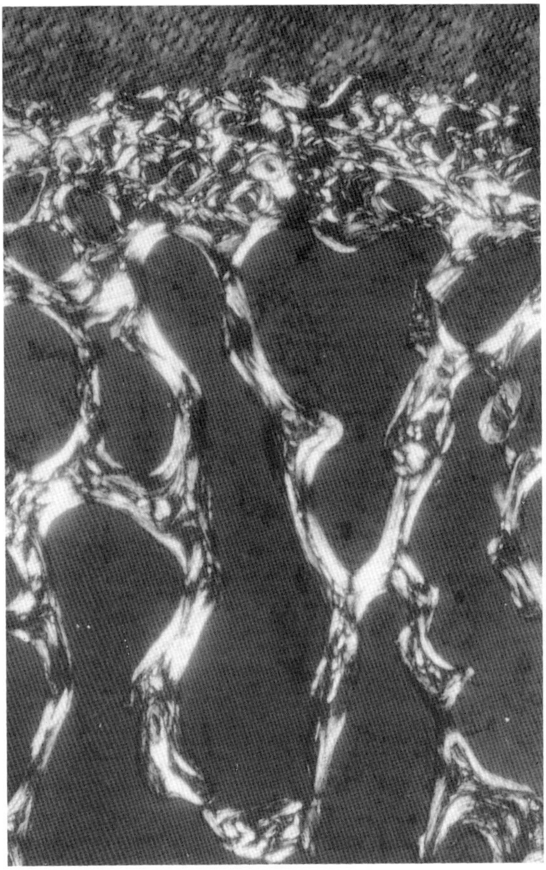

Fig. 24. Upper end of the arm bone in a 3-year-old pony. The inner part of the joint cartilage is at the top. Beneath this is the subchondral bone plate, which is supported by relatively thin bony bars, arranged perpendicularly. ×30, specimen exposed with polarized light.

v. *Epiphysis, metaphysis and diaphysis of long bones.* The growth plate is also referred to as the physis. The part of a long bone which is above (upper end of a long bone) or below (lower end of a long bone) and including the growth plate is called the epiphysis. The part of a long bone that is beyond the growth plate, the zone of trabeculae projecting from the growth plate, is called the metaphysis. The shaft of a long bone is called the diaphysis. The diaphysis is also called the cortex. Contained within the cortex is the marrow space, also called the medullary space. The shaft, thus, consists of bark and marrow.

The different parts of a long bone are named according to their relation to the growth plate; this is illustrated in Fig. 25. The specimen is the forearm bone of a 10-week-old thoroughbred filly.

4. Development of short bones

The ossification center of the short bones (the knee and the hock) appears much later than that of the shaft and at roughly the same time as that of the lower or upper end of long bones. Fig. 26 is a radiograph of the left knee of a 287-day-old fetus. The shaft of the forearm bone is in advanced development, and the ossification center of the lower end is in place, though its final shape has not yet been suggested. In the knee, there are 2 rows that will become short bones, 4 in the upper row and 3 in the lower. At the stage of fetal development shown in Fig. 26, only the ossification center of the outermost bone of the upper row (the accessory knee bone) has appeared. The remaining ossification centers appear from 290 to 330 days of fetal life. The situation is similar in the hock.

The ossification of the cartilage model starts in the center, and the events of conversion of cartilage into bone are the same as they are in long bones. The process moves peripherally, and at birth the final shape of a short bone is well established (Fig. 27). The section, from the front to the back end, is from the largest of the short bones of the upper row of knee bones (located in the middle and, therefore, called the intermediate knee bone). All but the most peripheral cartilage model has been converted into bone. The upper end, which plays against the forearm bone, and the lower end, which plays against the largest bone of the lower row (the third knee bone), will form a joint cartilage. This joint cartilage, in its mature state, appears as any joint cartilage of long bones as described above. The front and back ends of this short bone will be completely converted into bone to which the joint capsule will attach itself.

In the development of a short bone, a growth plate is not formed. This is the main difference between short and long bones. A long bone has growth plate(s), but a short bone does not. By that definition, the coffin bone is considered a short bone.

Fig. 25. Forearm bone of a 10-week-old thoroughbred filly. The bone has been cut from outside to inside at the thickest part. To the left is a picture of the cut surface, to the right a radiograph of a ¼-inch thick slab section cut parallel to the surface of the left section.

The large arrows (top and bottom, left figure) point to the joint cartilage, which is not seen in the radiograph (right). Inside the joint cartilage at both ends, is the epiphysis (E), seen grossly and in the radiograph. Inside the epiphysis is the growth plate, indicated by white arrow heads. The plate is greyish white in the gross specimen and presents a negative image in the radiograph, because it has no radiographic density. Inside the growth plate is the metaphysis, M in the figures. The shaft, or diaphysis, is indicated in the gross specimen and in the radiograph by thin arrows. Between the upper and lower metaphysis is the marrow cavity, indicated by C.

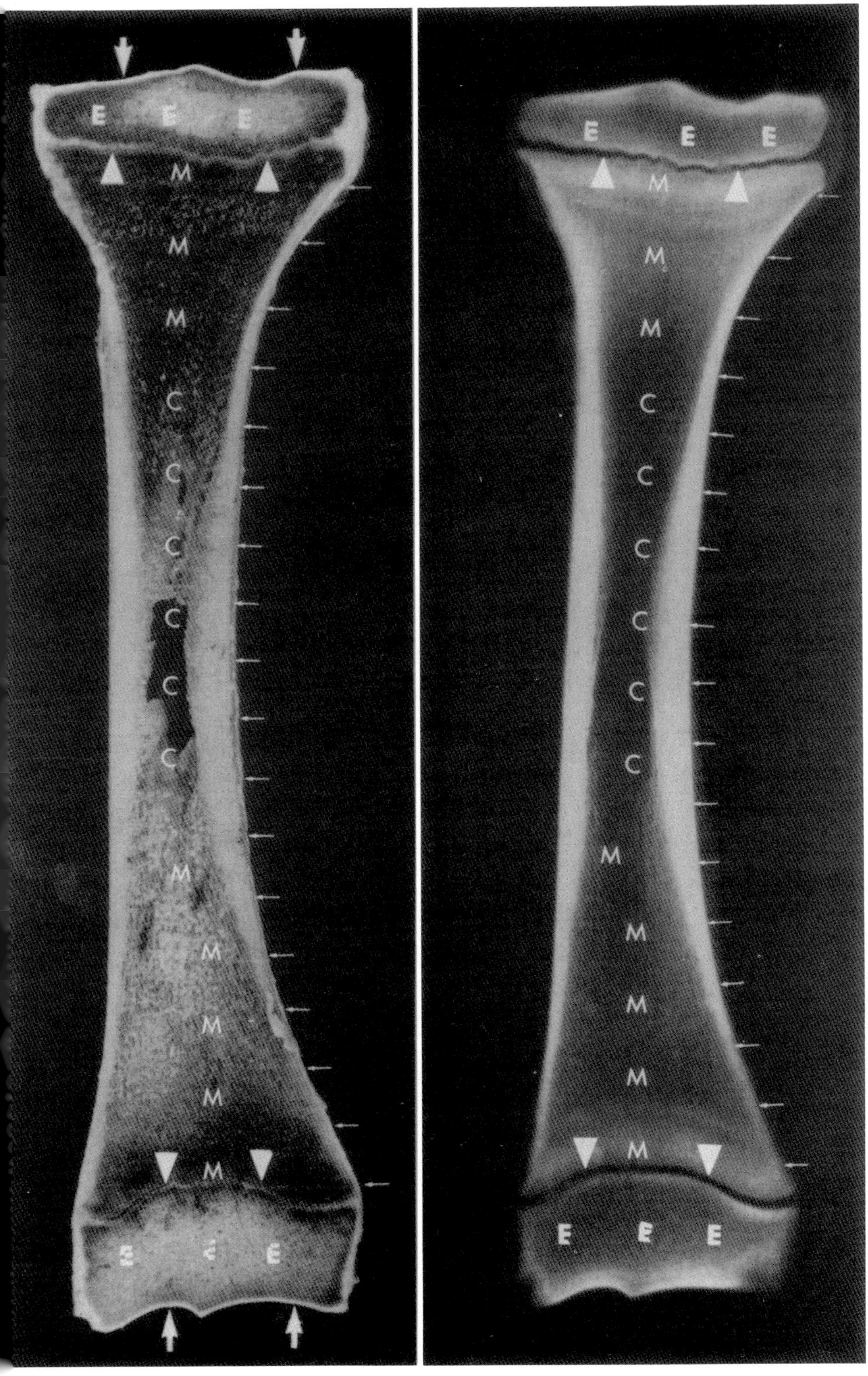
E E E
M
M
M
C
C
C
C
C
C
M
M
M
M
M
E E E
E E E
M
M
M
C
C
C
C
C
C
M
M
M
M
M
E E E

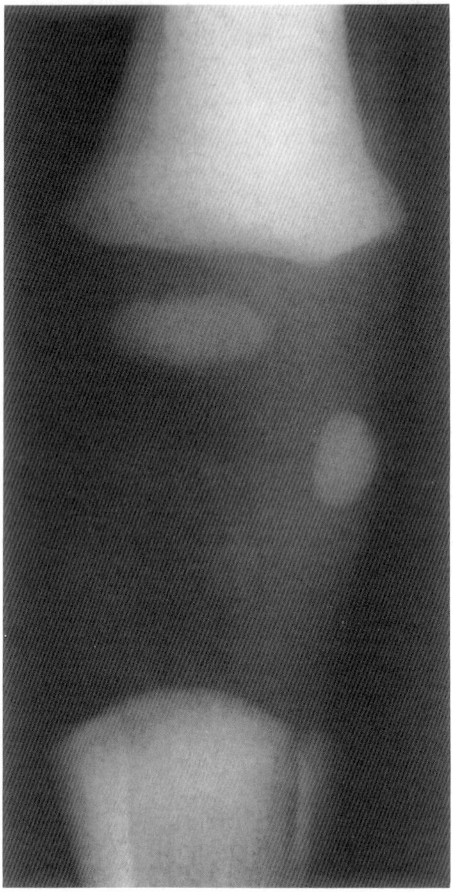

Fig. 26. Radiograph in front view of the knee region of a 287-day-old female thoroughbred fetus. At the top is the lower end of the forearm bone, which is well developed. The grey structure just beneath the shaft of the forearm bone is the ossification center of the lower end of the forearm bone. At the bottom is the top of the cannon bone. The area between the forearm bone and the cannon bone is the knee region. Only one ossification center of the seven knee bones has appeared at this fetal age: the grey area to the right represents the ossification center of the accessory knee bone.

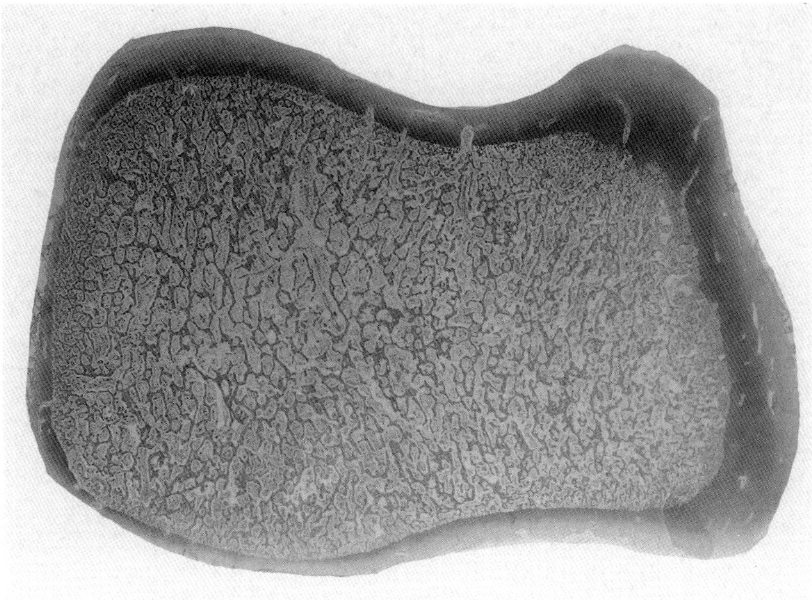

Fig. 27. Microscopic section of the middle knee bone of the upper row (intermediate knee bone). The upper end is the surface that plays against the lower end of the forearm bone, front end is to the right. The specimen is from a newborn thoroughbred colt. The final shape of the bone has been established. Most of the field is occupied by bony bars. The cartilage remains in all four surfaces of the bone. ×3.3.

5. Development of flat bones

The shoulder blade is the only flat bone of the limbs. The shoulder blade develops from four ossification centers: one for the upper end and three for the lower end. The center for the upper end appears at age 9 to 12 months of the foal. The lower ones develop in the fetus and are well established at birth. In Fig. 28, the ossification centers are shown in a 2½-week-old thoroughbred filly foal. The ossification center of the body, which appears in the 60-to-70-day old fetus, has formed the body, including most of the joint area. The ossification center of the front end of the joint area, which appears shortly before birth, is likewise well defined. The front end of the lower part of the shoulder blade comes from an ossification center that first appears in the 140-to-170-day-old fetus, is likewise in an advanced stage of development. The union of the three ossification centers of the lower shoulder blade occurs at about one year of age, and the union of the upper end with the body occurs at about three years of age.

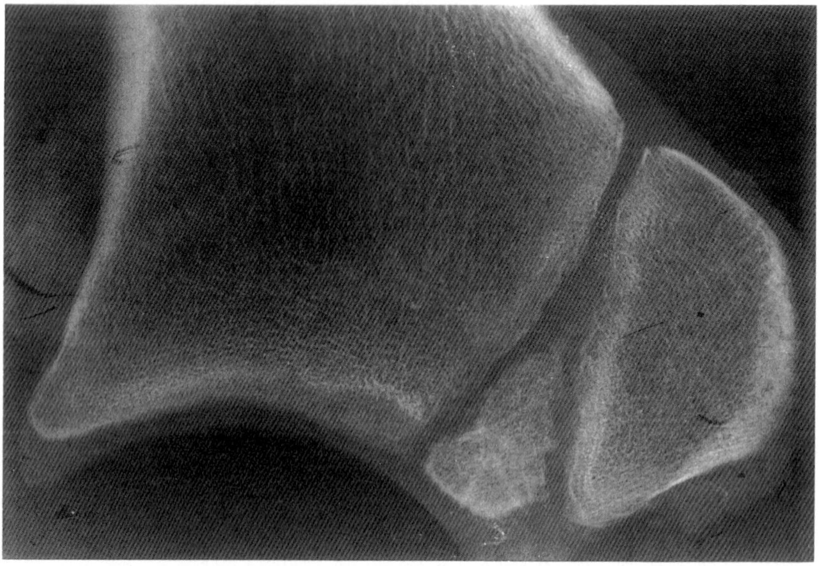

Fig. 28. Radiograph of a slab section of the lower end of the shoulder blade. Front end is to the right. The specimen is from a 2½-week-old thoroughbred filly.

The largest unit (middle, left, upper) is the body of the shoulder blade with the neck at top. It is well advanced at this age, and the joint area is well established. The small triangular part forms the front end of the joint area. The ossification center to the right is forming the front end of the lower part of the shoulder blade; this is the point of origin of the muscle that bends the elbow joint.

At this age, the ossification centers are well established. The ossification center of the upper part of the shoulder blade, which is formed at age 9 to 12 months of the foal, is not included in the picture.

6. Development of sesamoid bones

Sesamoid bones, as defined in Chapter II, are bones that develop within tendons. They form, develop, and mature just as the short bones do.

IV. OSTEOCHONDROSIS

The word osteochondrosis (OCH), which has no popular counterpart, means a non-inflammatory condition involving bone and cartilage (Greek osteo = bone + chondros = cartilage + -osis, a word ending indicating a non-inflammatory process).

In Chapter III, we stressed that all limb bones develop from cartilage. The normal development requires normal nutrition of the mare and the growing foal, normal hormonal activities, normal everything. If these requirements are not present, the conversion of cartilage into bone goes wrong. In the simplest terms, we define OCH as the FAILURE OF CARTILAGE TO CONVERT INTO BONE.

Conversion of cartilage into bone occurs in the developing fetus and during growth after birth. OCH can, accordingly, develop only during these stages. It can persist in the mature horse, but once maturity has been reached, OCH will no longer develop.

OCH is, as we will describe in future chapters, a major reason why young horses and racing horses break down. We will begin with a general description of the many manifestations of this disease.

1. Retained cartilage

Retained cartilage simply means that a chunk of cartilage did not participate in the conversion into bone. This can occur in any bone. In the long bones, it occurs mainly in the ends, and in short bones, beneath the joint cartilage.

Fig. 29 presents the upper surface of the lower row of knee bones in a 1½-year-old thoroughbred colt. In the fourth knee bone there is a pin-point defect in the cartilage (a). It looks innocent from the surface, but a section through this defect (b) reveals a large chunk of cartilage within the bone. The radiograph of this slab section shows no mineral density (c). Obviously, this area is a weak point in the bone, a weakness which makes it prone to a fracture.

2. Cysts

A cyst results from death of retained cartilage.

Fig. 30, from the upper end of the arm bone of a 4-year-old thor-

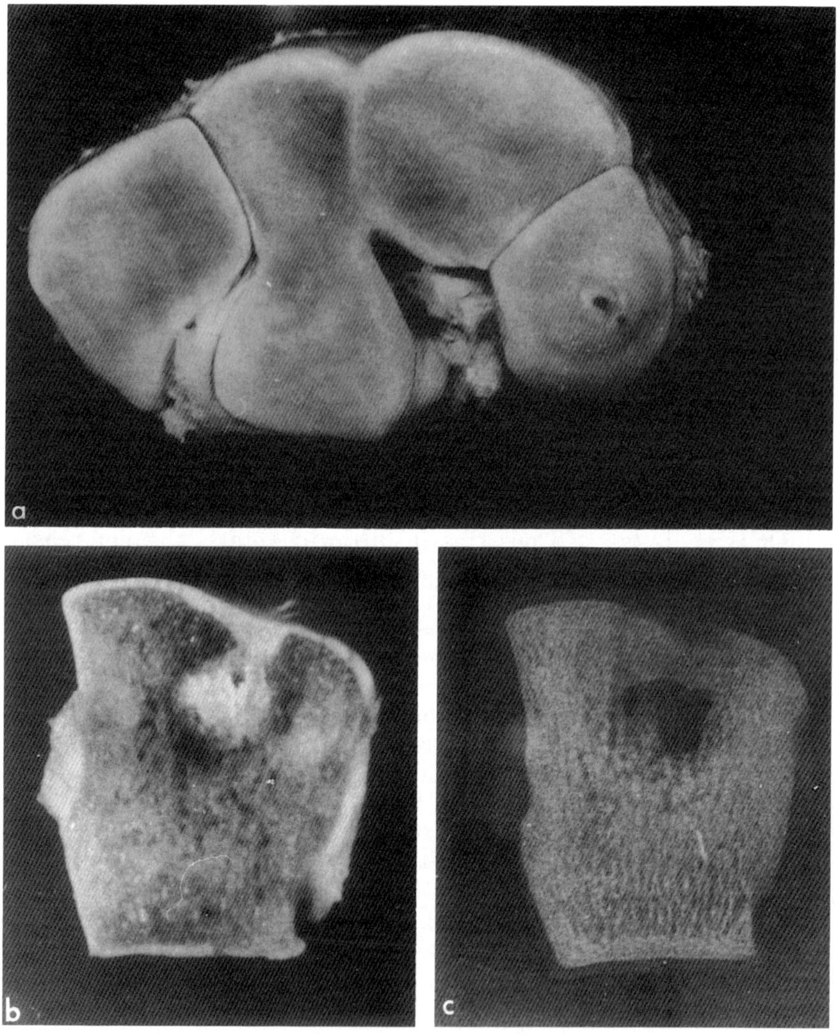

Fig. 29. Thoroughbred colt, 1.5-years-old. a shows the upper end of the lower row of knee bones. In the fourth knee bone to the right is a pin-point defect in the joint cartilage. A section through this defect appears in b. A large chunk of cartilage (white) is retained within the bone. c is a radiograph of the slab section in b. The retained cartilage shows minimal radiographic density.

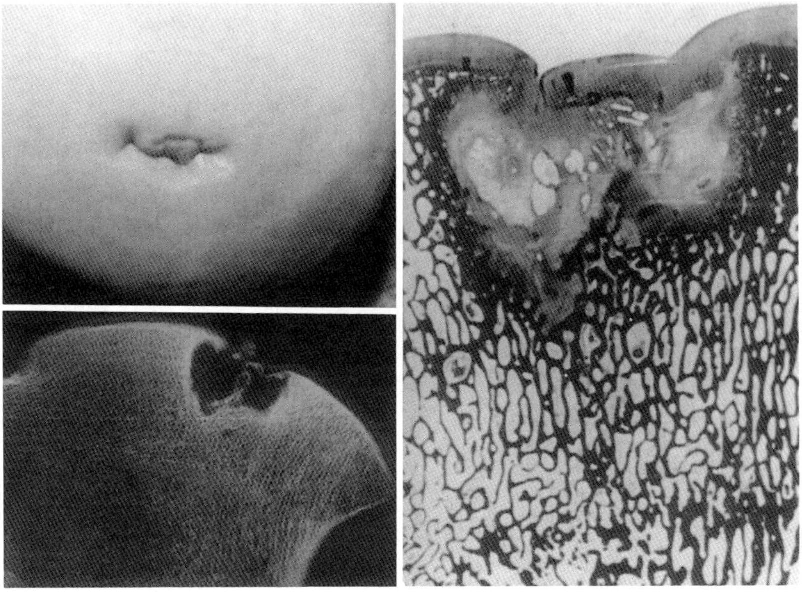

Fig. 30. Thoroughbred gelding, 4-year-old. Upper end of the right arm bone. In the upper left part is a large in-folded area of the cartilage. A radiograph of a slab section through this defect is shown in the lower left. There are deep cysts in the head of the arm bone. To the right is a microscopic section through the cysts. The center of the cysts is occupied by dying cartilage cells. The black material surrounding the cysts is retained cartilage. The cartilage above the cysts is caved in. ×4.

oughbred gelding, shows a large in-folded defect in the cartilage (upper left). A radiograph of a slab section through this defect shows a huge cyst which goes deep into the head of the arm bone (lower left). Under low-power microscopic magnification (right), we see that the cysts have been formed from dead, retained cartilage. The horse was, indeed, running on this bad bone. He fractured the left front sesamoid bones. The picture is included here to show the generalized nature of OCH in the skeleton.

A bone cyst can be most convincingly demonstrated in a microradiograph of a bone section. The section in Fig. 31 is from the upper end of the arm bone of a 4-year-old thoroughbred colt. The cyst has no microradiographic density and is lined by a thin layer of dense bone. In the same picture, we see a deep ditch extending into the bone beneath the joint cartilage. This ditch indicates a failure of cartilage to convert into bone. Note that cartilage does not show in a microradiograph.

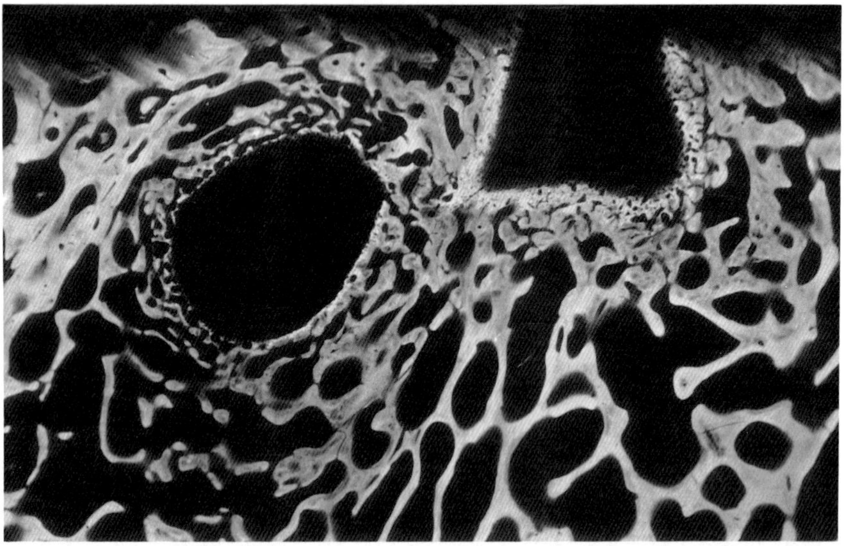

Fig. 31. Thoroughbred colt, 4-year-old. Upper end of the right arm bone. In the upper left part of this microradiograph is a cyst with no density. The cyst wall is comprised by a thin but dense layer of bone. In the upper right part is a "ditch" in the upper end of the bone. Again, this is caused by cartilage that failed to produce bone in that area. ×10.

3. Transverse trabeculation

In Chapter III we emphasized that the trabeculae of the epiphysis are normally arranged perpendicularly to the joint cartilage with its subchondral bone plate. When growth of the joint cartilage stops for one reason or the other, bone is laid down along the inner side of the cartilage; this bone is arranged transversely. When growth is resumed, this transverse bone will be pushed into the epiphysis and will appear in the radiograph, the microradiograph, and the microscopic section as a transverse trabecula. This is illustrated in Fig. 32, a microscopic section.

The same processes can also occur in the growth plate. The microradiographic expression of such transverse trabeculation is illustrated in Fig. 33.

Transverse trabeculation means that there has been a stop-and-go activity in the joint cartilage or in the growth plate. This is yet another manifestation of OCH.

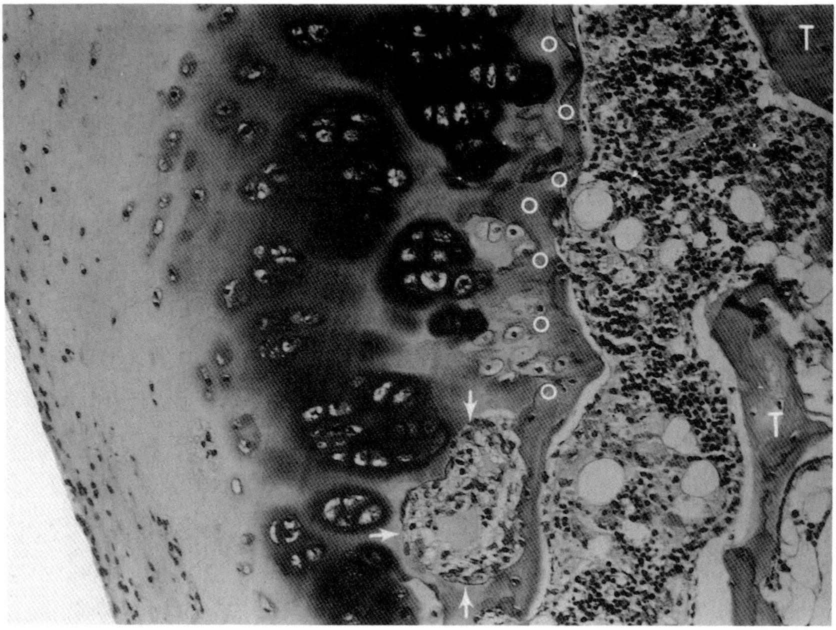

Fig. 32. Thoroughbred colt, 7-month-old. This is a section of the joint area of the elbow bone. Cartilage growth is minimal. The structure indicated by open circles is bone laid down horizontally along the inner part of the cartilage. In the area within arrows in the lower part, growth has resumed, at least to some extent. The bony bars labeled T are transversely arranged trabeculae. ×160.

4. Osteochondrosis dissecans

The world dissecans means "to cut up." The term osteochondrosis dissecans (OCD) means an osteochondrosis in which a part of the cartilage, with or without bone, has been separated from the main bone.

OCD is illustrated in Figs. 34-39, all from the lower end of the thigh bone of a yearling thoroughbred colt.

In Fig. 34 is the lower end of the thigh bone. In the lateral trochlea, a large part of the cartilage is separated from the main bone. It has been separated away, the very definition of OCD. We now move to Fig. 35 in which slab sections parallel to the dissecting process are shown. The upper part of that picture shows that the dissecting change can occur within the cartilage and the lower part shows that it can occur between cartilage and bone. Wherever it occurs, it is still a dissecting change. The radiographs of the slab sections shown in Fig. 34 are shown in Fig. 36. It is noteworthy that there are cysts inside the cartilage, and that the bone beneath the cartilage is denser than normal.

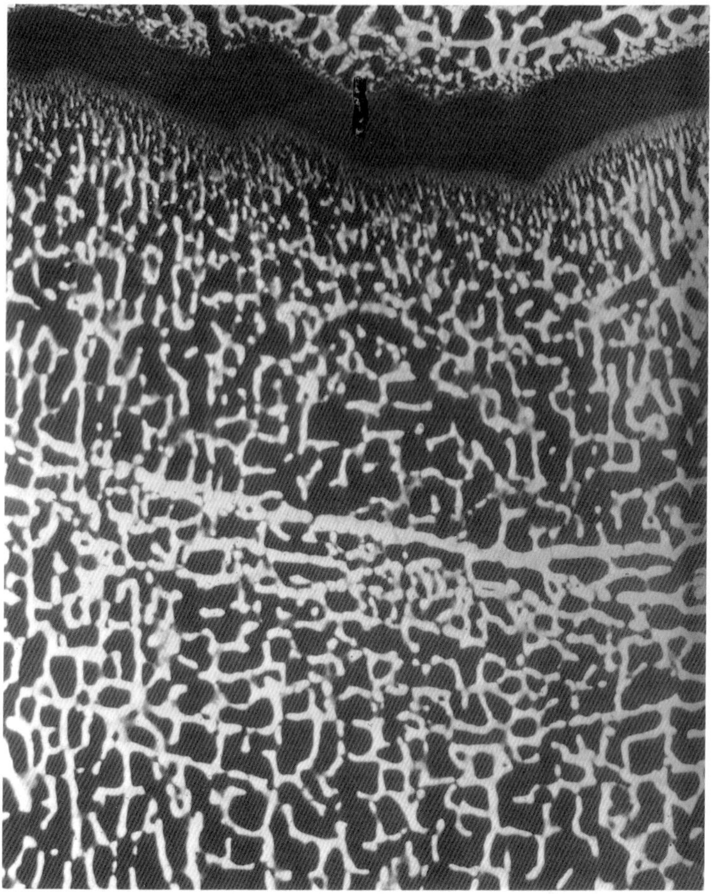

Fig. 33. Same horse as in Fig. 32. This is a microradiograph of the upper part of the forearm. The black band at the top is the growth plate—the cartilage does not show in a microradiograph. In the middle of the picture is a thick, white line which represents a transversely-laid-down bone at the growth plate some time ago. It has now been pushed down deep into the bone, but it tells you that, some time ago, the growth plate failed to grow. ×3.6.

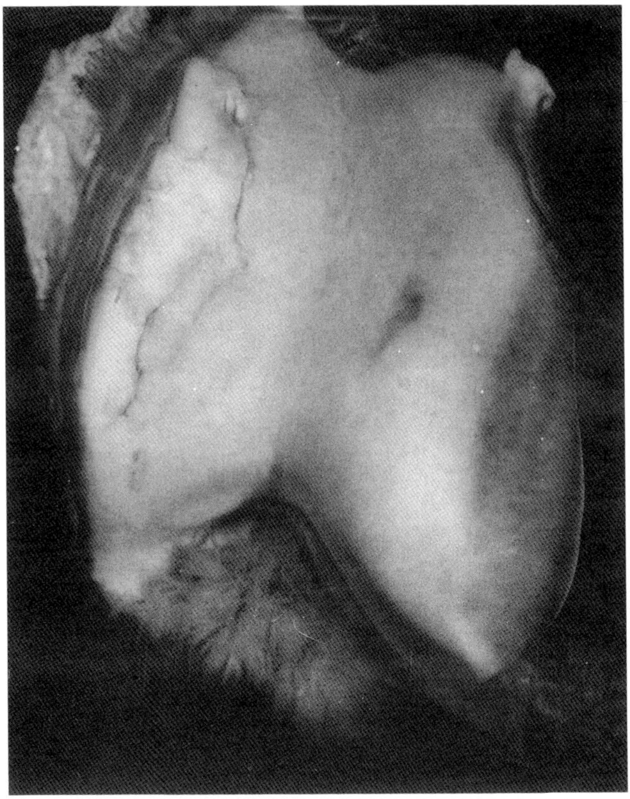

Figs. 34-39. These are from the lower end of the thigh bone of a yearling thoroughbred colt.

Fig. 34. This picture shows the gross appearance of osteochondrosis dissecans (OCD) in the lateral trochlea.

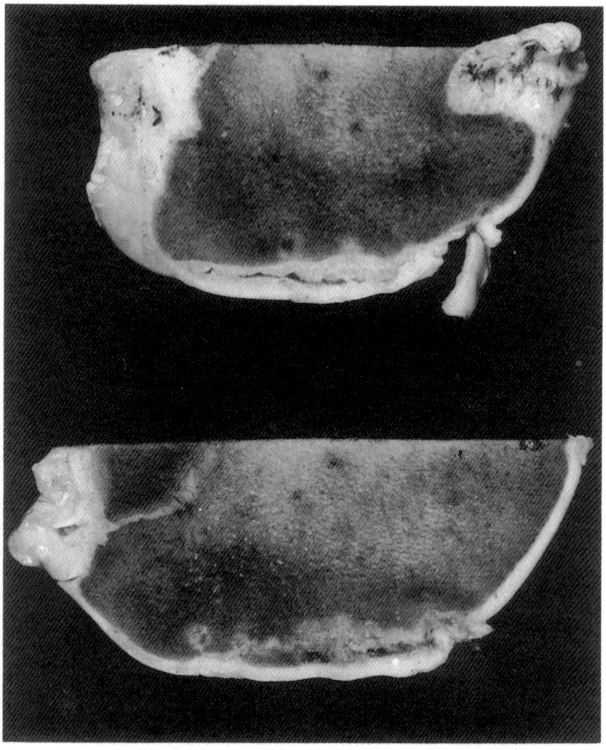

Fig. 35. These are slab sections parallel to and including the OCD shown in Fig. 34. In the upper part, the dissecting change occurs *within* the cartilage. In the lower part, the dissecting change occurs between cartilage and bone.

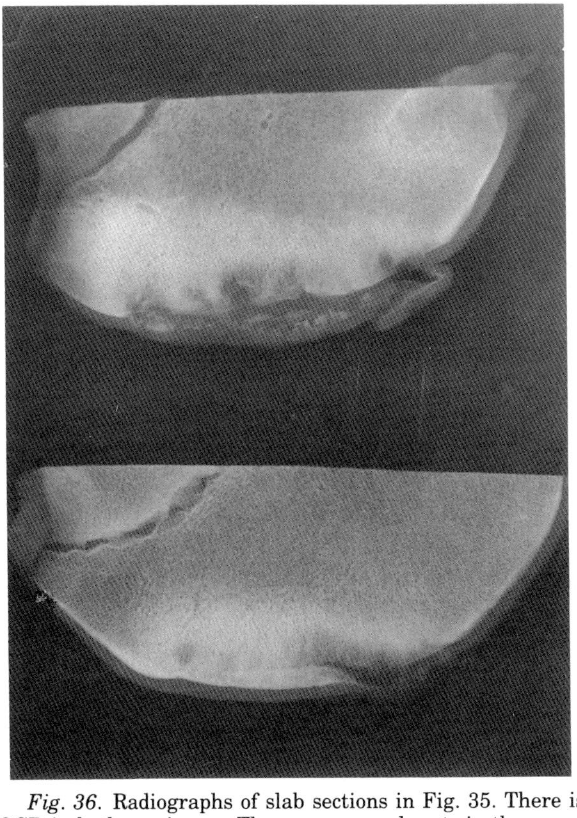

Fig. 36. Radiographs of slab sections in Fig. 35. There is OCD in both specimens. There are several cysts in the upper specimen. Note that the bone beneath the cartilage is denser than normal.

We now go to the microscope to find what is happening. We see in Fig. 37 that the gap is occurring within the cartilage and that undifferentiated cartilage is projecting into the epiphysis, where we would

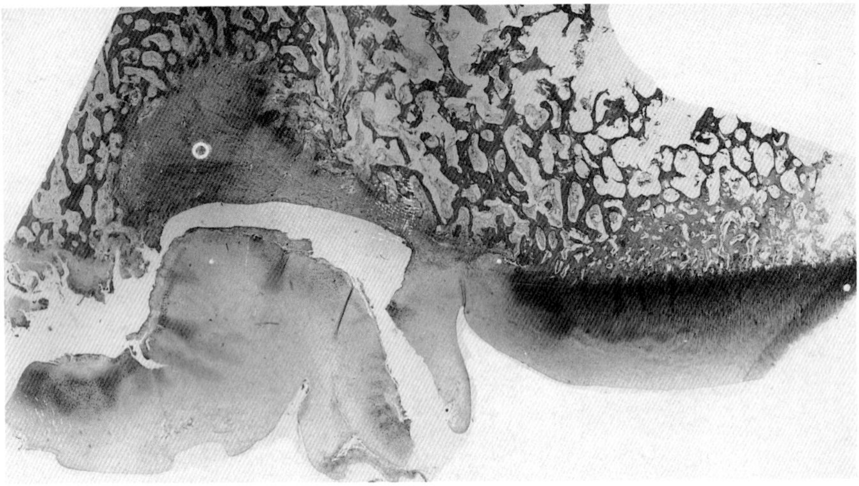

Fig. 37. This is a microscopic section through one of the slabs in Figs. 35. The dissection occurs *within* the cartilage. The open circle in the picture is in the center of a piece of cartilage that did not convert into bone. ×6.5.

have expected bone. In Fig. 38, bone tissue has started to develop within cartilage, but the cartilage facing the epiphysis does not produce bone. Figures 35 and 36 are eloquent demonstrations of our definitions of OCH: a failure of cartilage to convert into bone.

The cartilage changes demonstrated in the previous figures are not restricted to joint cartilages. The same thing can also occur in growth plates. This is illustrated in Fig. 39. The picture concerns the growth plate of the lower end of the thigh bone of the horse in the six previous pictures. The cartilage does not function, large areas of undifferentiated cartilage are retained on the back of the growth plate. Further evidence of previous malfunction of the plate is the transverse trabeculation in the metaphysis.

5. "Chip Fractures"

A commonly diagnosed disorder of bones, especially of the upper front end of the long pastern bone, is "chip fracture." This term is, as we will show in pictures, a misnomer. It is not a fracture.

A very common finding in thoroughbred race horses is a bulging of the cartilage at the upper front end of the long pastern bone (Fig. 40a). Sections from the front to the back have been made through this bulging cartilage and pictures of these slabs are presented in the same figure (b). A small ossification center appears at the very top of the front end of the long pastern bone. This little piece of bone is black in

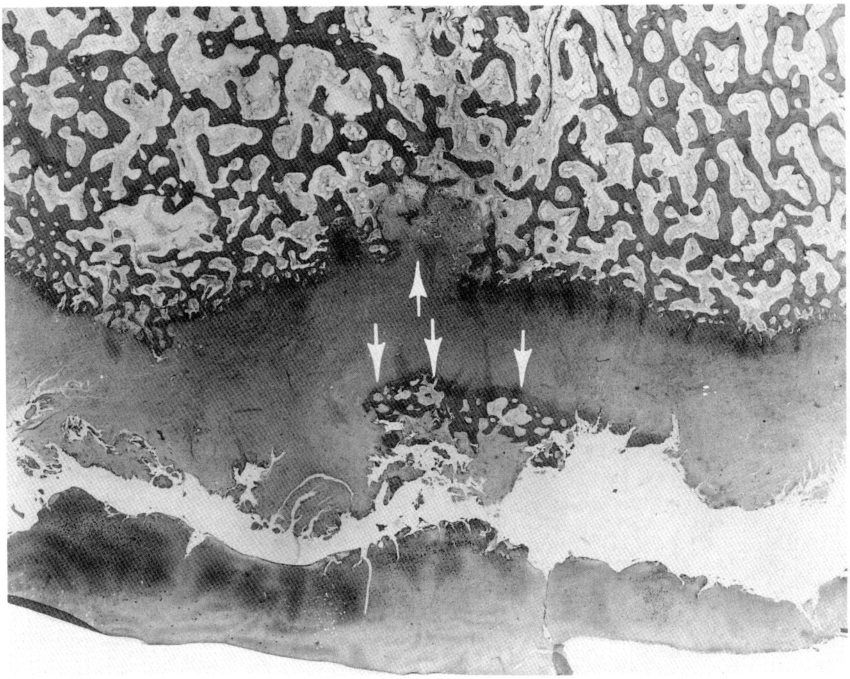

Fig. 38. Another microscopic section through one of the slabs in Fig. 35. The dissection, again, occurs within the cartilage. In front of the arrows pointing down is an area of bone formation within the cartilage. At the arrow pointing up is a chunk of cartilage that did not form bone. ×6.5.

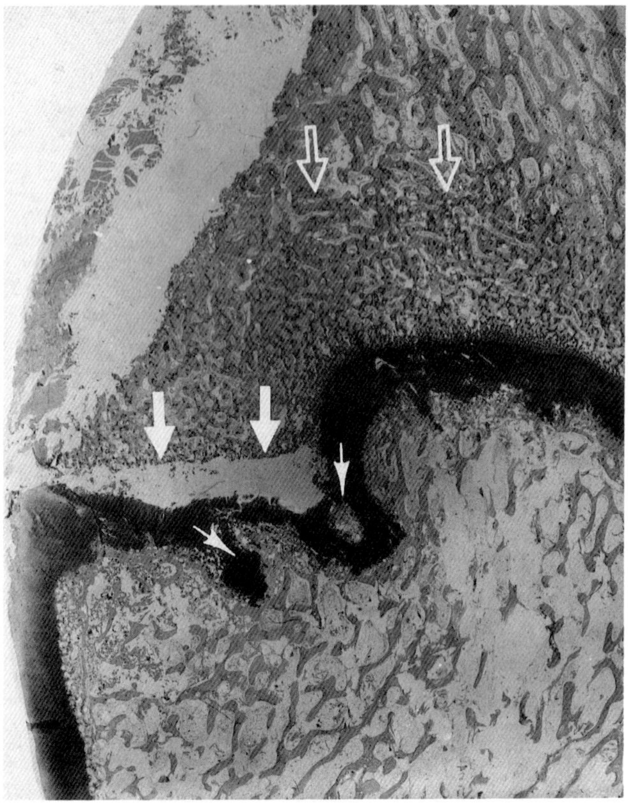

Fig. 39. Same horse as in Fig. 35. The section is from the lower end of the thigh bone. The black horizontal line is the growth plate. There is a wide separation between the growth plate and the bone at the filled arrows. In front of the small arrows are chunks of cartilage that were left behind in the process of converting cartilage into bone. At the open large arrows are transversely arranged trabeculae. ×24.

the picture. Between that little piece of bone and the main bone, the long pastern bone, is a white structure, which is cartilage. Thus, the little piece of bone is held in position by cartilage. In others words, there is no fracture.

In the lower right part of the same picture (c) are radiographs of the slab section. These are the typical radiographic pictures of what is commonly called a chip fracture. If you now compare these radiographs with the gross pictures, you will appreciate the fact that this is *not* a chip fracture. It is a type of OCH.

A microradiograph of the slab section in Fig. 40b, upper part, is shown in Fig. 41. The little piece of bone to the left has not joined the main bone to the right but is held in place by cartilage, the black area between the bones. Fig. 42 represents the same area of another horse, and the picture shows that the separation between the two pieces could not possibly be a chip. The facing bone surfaces present concavities which could not, under any circumstances, occur in a fracture. Fig. 43 shows the similar situation, but in this case, the gap is far narrower though still there. Finally, in Fig. 44, the pieces, if there were any, have joined to form one common unit. We emphasize that the main bone, the long pastern bone, in these figures (41-44) shows denser than normal bone. This is referred to as osteopetrosis (too much bone tissue per volume of bone or rock solid bone).

The microradiographs presented in Figs. 41-43 clearly show that what is usually referred to as chip fracture is not at all a fracture but an expression of OCH. To further emphasize this point, a microscopic picture is presented in Fig. 45. The upper front end of the long pastern bone in this 4-year-old thoroughbred colt shows a large chunk of cartilage. Within this cartilage are two small ossification centers. The bone in these centers is not connected to the main bone, but the centers are held in position by the retained cartilage. Again, the main bone is very dense.

6. Joint mouse

If a piece of cartilage with or without bone is actually detached, it becomes free in the joint space and is referred to as a joint mouse. The front limb sesamoid bones of a 3½-year-old thoroughbred gelding are shown in Fig. 46. The left fetlock joint contained a free-floating mouse of impressive size. It was ½ inch long and about ¼ inch wide and thick. It has been pinned to its site of origin in Fig. 46, that is, to the upper end of the inner left sesamoid bone. The outer sesamoid bone of the left limb shows a deep ditch in the cartilage. This is an instance of OCH, and presumably such a change in the cartilage and bone preceded the detachment of the joint mouse in the inner sesamoid bone.

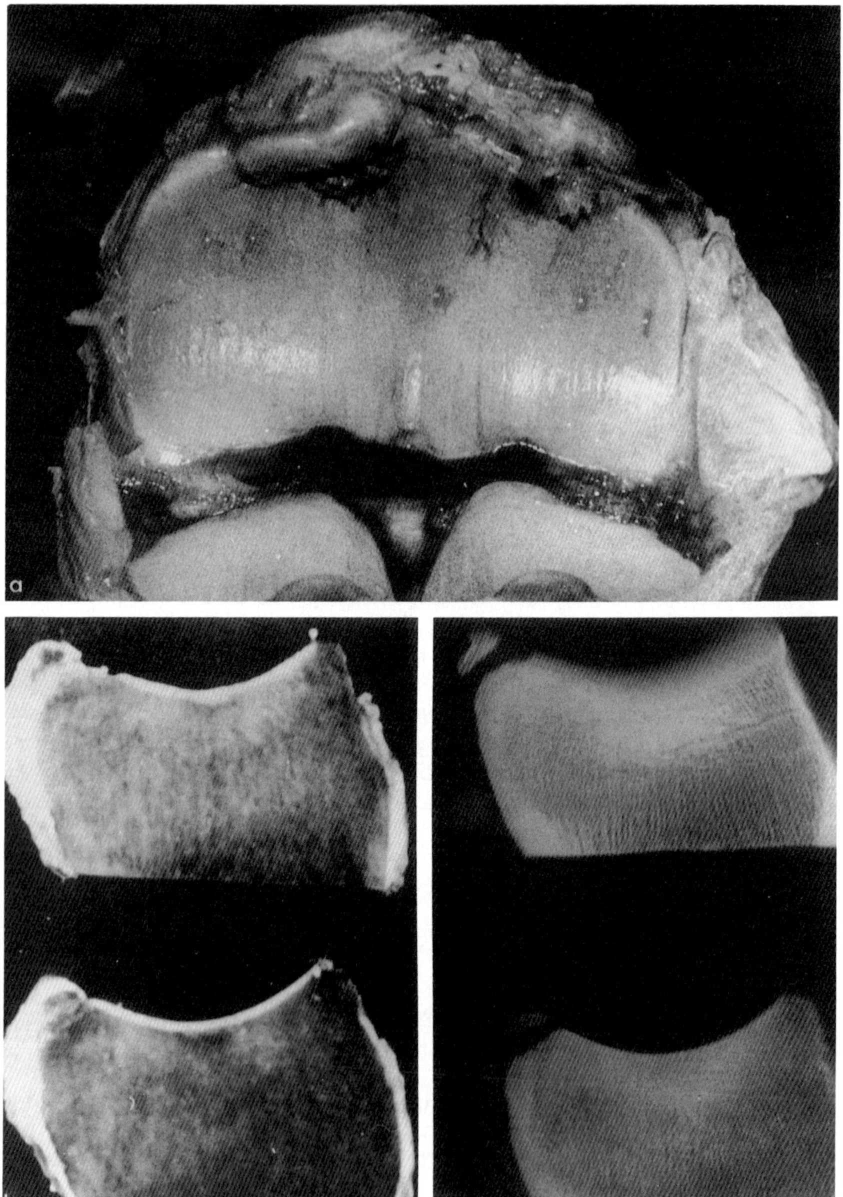
a
b
c

The shape of the right sesamoid bones is about normal, but great irregularities in the cartilage suggest OCH.

We now take the joint mouse under the microscope (Fig. 47) and find that, except for small areas at both ends, the mouse is covered by cartilage of varying thickness. Within the cartilage is an area where the cartilage grew independently of the surrounding cartilage. A large tongue of cartilage projected into the mouse and the bone bars are arranged haphazardly with no defined purpose. This is OCH in the joint mouse, and OCH is exactly the reason for it becoming a joint mouse.

The above examples of OCH will suffice here. There are more variants, to which we will return in the next chapter.

The descriptions and illustrations of OCH in this chapter show that the changes can occur, on gross examination, just about anywhere in the limb bones. Upon microscopic examination of grossly normal cartilage and bone, similar but less advanced changes occur everywhere. OCH is, thus, a generalized disease of the skeleton, but its gross manifestations vary greatly in site and degree. If you find a joint mouse or infolded cartilage with a cyst beneath, or a pin-point defect in the cartilage with a chunk of cartilage retained beneath, you will find, under the microscope, similar but less advanced changes elsewhere in the skeleton.

Fig. 40. Thoroughbred filly, 3-year-old. In a (top) is the upper end of the right long pastern bone. The front end shows a large bulging of the cartilage to the left. To the right in the same picture is a big defect, which may represent the detachment of such bulging cartilage.

In b (lower left) are slab sections through the bulging cartilage of a, left part. The front end is to the left. The dark spot at the upper left corner represents bone. The white material between that spot and the main bone is cartilage. The bone spot is, thus, still attached to the main bone.

Part c of the picture presents radiographs of the slab sections in b. There is a gap between the small bone spots at the upper front end of the main bone. The cartilage connection between the two bone pieces is not shown in the radiographs.

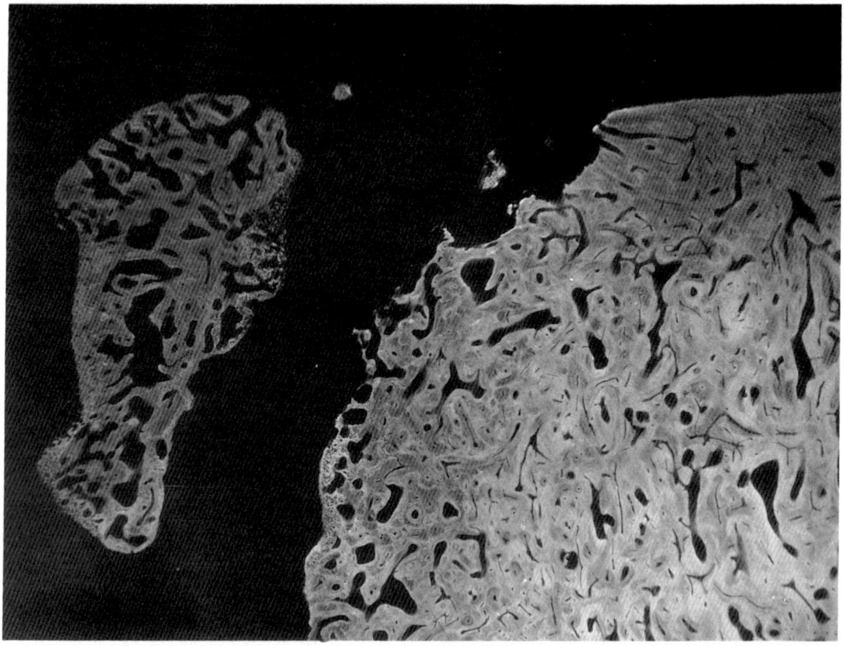

Fig. 41. This is a microradiograph of the upper slab section in Fig. 40, b and c. To the left is an ossification center that has not joined the main bone. The black area between the ossification center at the upper left and the main bone is cartilage, which does not show in a microradiograph. Note that there is severely increased density of the main bone. ×10.

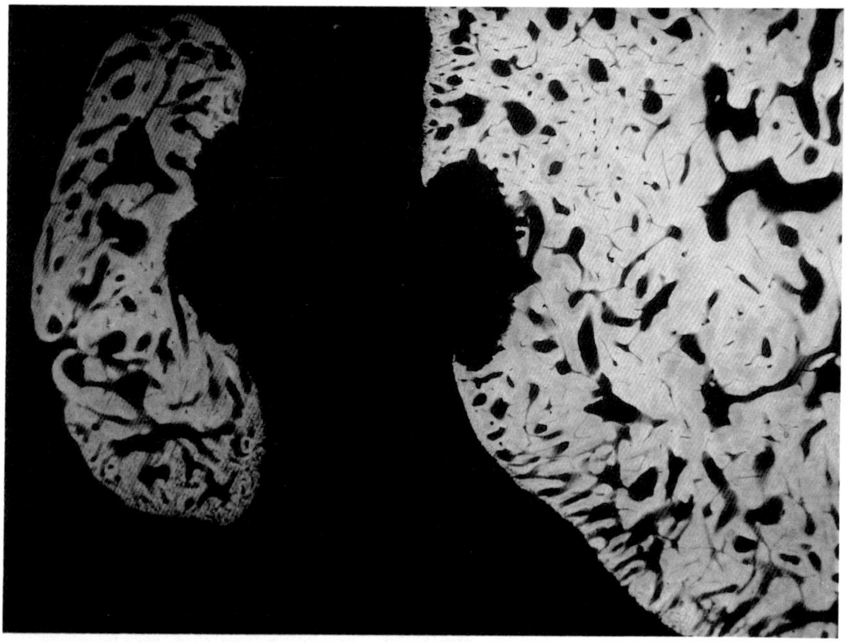

Fig. 42. Thoroughbred colt, ½-year-old. Microradiograph of the upper front end of the long pastern bone, orientation as in Fig. 41.

The message of this picture is much the same as that of Fig. 41, but with an additional feature. Note that the facing surfaces of the bone piece to the left and of the main bone show concavities. This could not possibly occur in a fracture. Again, note the increased density of the main long pastern bone. ×10.

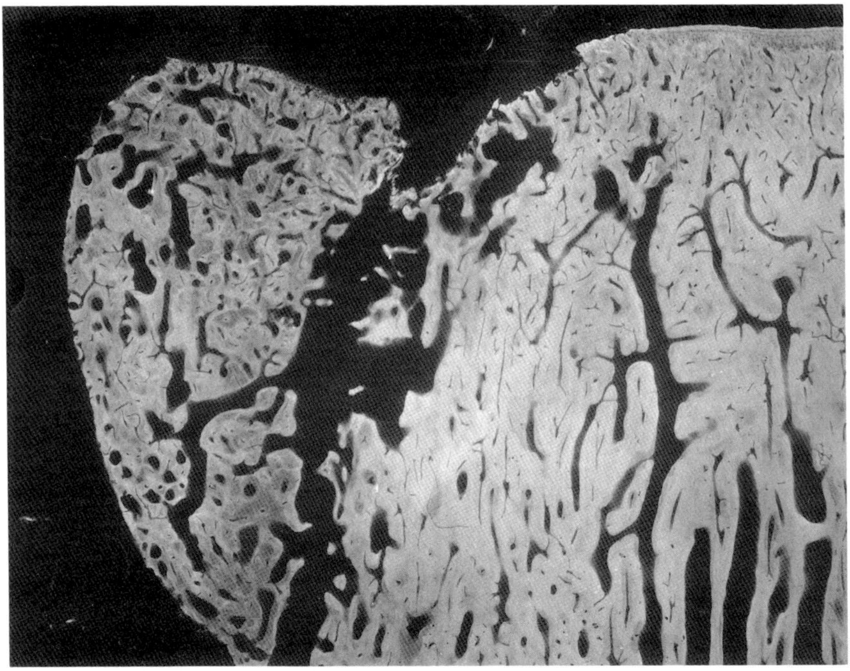

Fig. 43. Thoroughbred colt, 4-year-old. Microradiograph of a specimen as in Fig. 41. The ossification center to the left is now much closer to the main bone, but fusion has not occurred. The main bone is very dense. ×10.

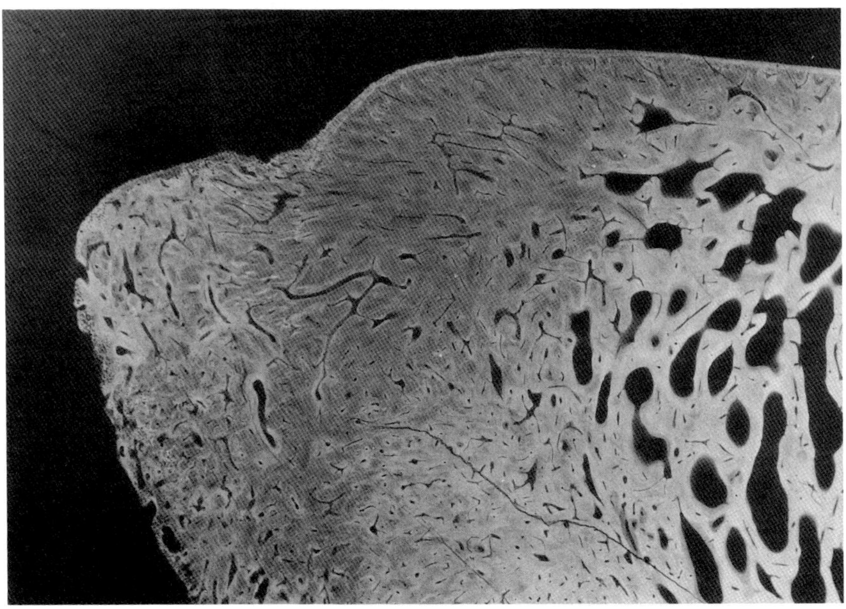

Fig. 44. Thoroughbred stallion, 5-year-old. Microradiograph of specimen as in Fig. 41. The picture presents a solid area of the upper front end of the long pastern bone. Again, note the impressive density of that part of the long pastern bone. ×10.

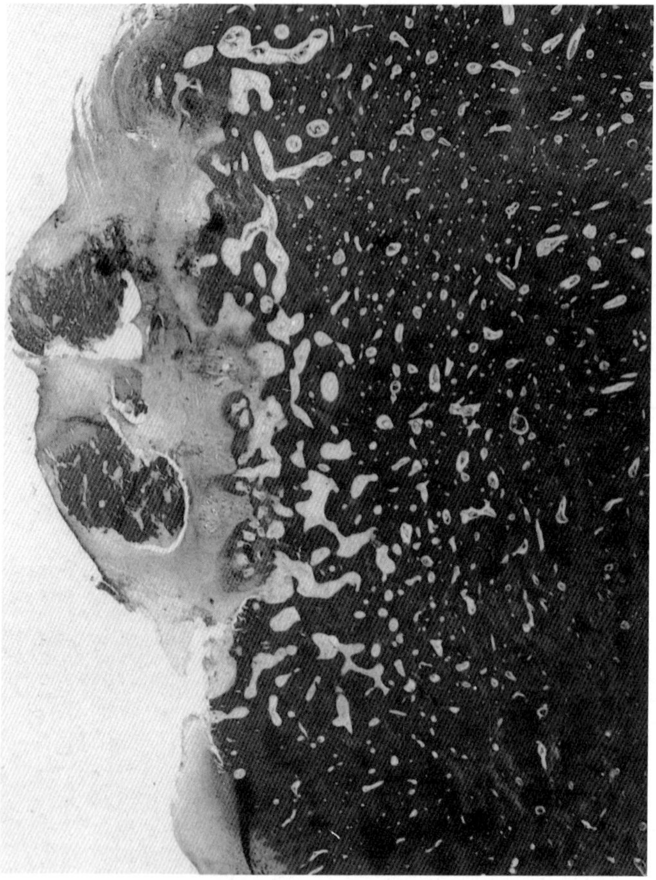

Fig. 45. Thoroughbred colt, 4-year-old. The figure shows the upper front end of the long pastern bone under low microscopic magnification. The grey area at the left center and upper part represents cartilage. Within this cartilage are two independent ossification centers (dark areas), which have not joined the main bone to the right. Note that these two ossification centers are separated from the main bone by cartilage. ×9.5.

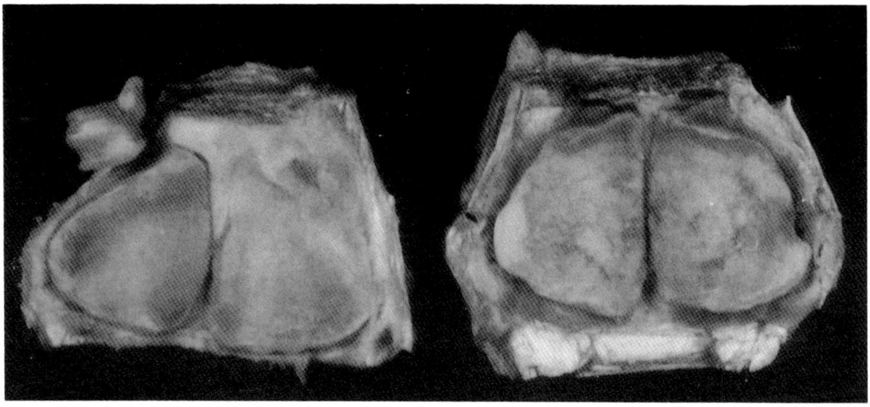

Fig. 46. Thoroughbred gelding, 3½-year-old. The picture shows the sesamoid bones of the front limbs. The inner sesamoid bone of the left limb is to the far left. A large joint mouse has been pinned to its origin at the upper left corner of the left inner sesamoid bone. The outer sesamoid bone of that limb shows a deep grove almost separating the corner from the main bone. The right front limb bone sesamoids show severe osteochondrosis (OCH).

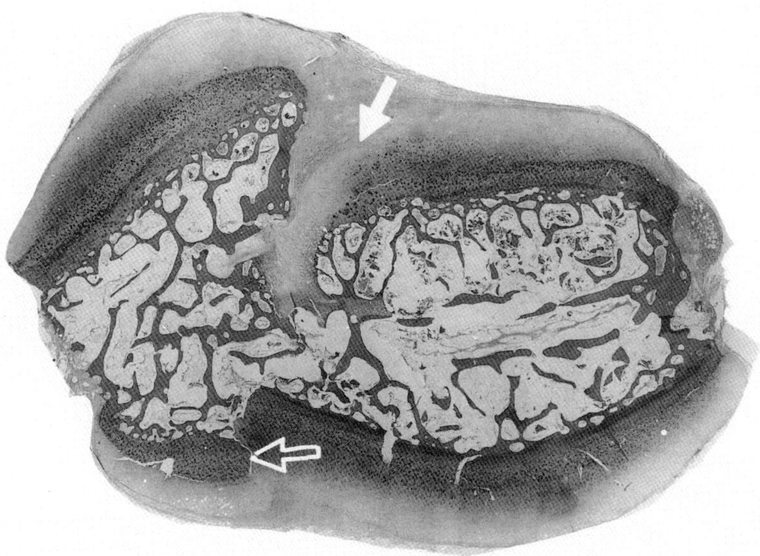

Fig. 47. This is a microscopic section of the joint mouse in Fig. 46. The mouse has a cartilage cover, except at the ends to the left and right. The picture shows severe OCH within the detached piece. In front of the open arrow is a well-demarcated area of cartilage that grew independently of the surrounding cartilage. In front of the solid arrow at top is a wide peninsula of cartilage that projects deep into the specimen. The bone bars of the joint mouse are arranged haphazardly. ×8.

V. SOME THAT DID NOT MAKE IT

Relatively few of all horses bred for racing ever race. There is, to our knowledge, no statistical information why this happens to racing horses in the U.S. Information on this subject in British thoroughbred horses is available (1). Of 6,530 foals born in 1975 eligible for training, only 47% trained at 2 years of age, 51% at 3 years and 38% at four years of age. The percentages of horses that raced were lower: 2-year-olds 43%, 3-year-olds 41% and 4-year-olds 22%. The report did not address the question of why this is the case.

This poor performance of eligible horses together with failure of mares to conceive, abortions, and non-surviving foals, added up to 73% "wastage" in thoroughbred horses from conception to 4 years of age. The cumulative financial losses for the 1974 season were calculated to be more than 15 million pounds sterling.

In this chapter, we will give a few reasons why foals bred for racing did not make it. We can give no figures on how common these conditions are. The cases to be described are horses submitted to the Veterinary Hospital at Cornell University for examination or donated as hopeless cases. We are thus dealing with a highly selected material.

In Chapter IV we presented pictures (Figs. 34-39) of a yearling thoroughbred colt with severe OCH in the thigh bone. Resulting lameness prevented training this colt. The illustrations (Figs. 46 and 47) of a joint mouse in a 3½-year-old thoroughbred gelding show another reason why the horse never raced.

1. "Contracted tendons"

A thoroughbred filly, 5 months and 20 days old, was donated to the College of Veterinary Medicine, two months before the picture in Fig. 48 was taken. The reason for donation was "contracted tendons" of the filly's front limbs. It was not stated at what age that diagnosis was made.

A close look at this picture will reveal that the diagnosis is wrong. Had there been a contraction of the flexor tendons, all joints from the knee and down would have been flexed (that is, bent backwards). The fetlock joints are, however, extended (that is, bent forwards). Had the tendons been contracted, the fetlock joint would also have been flexed,

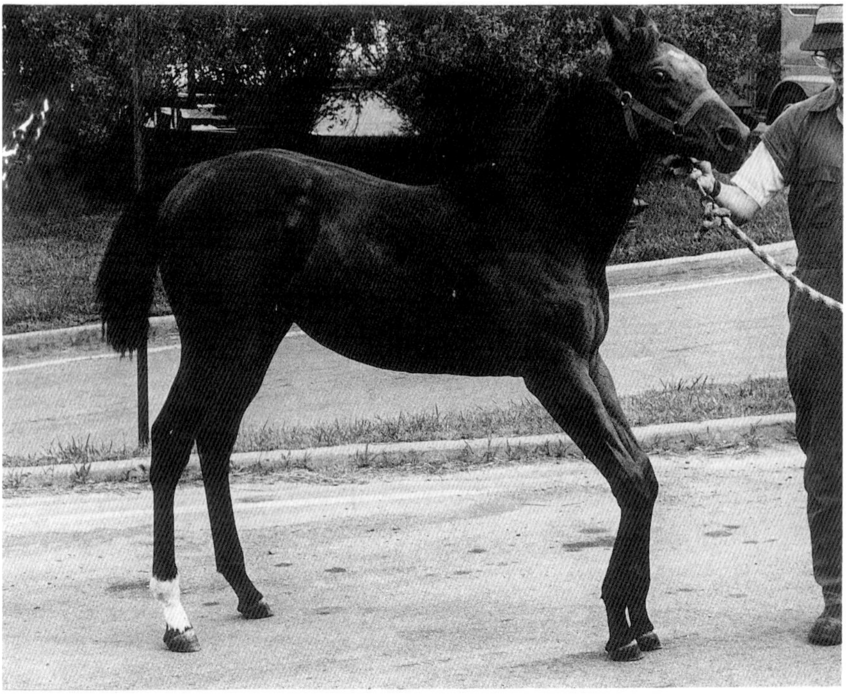

Fig. 48. Thoroughbred filly, 5 months and 20 days old. The knees are flexed, and the fetlock joints are extended.

not extended. The deep flexor tendons attaches to the back side of the coffin bone and a "contracted" deep flexor tendon would have flexed the fetlock joint.

The upper view of the lower row of knee bones is shown in Fig. 49. The back end of the middle knee bone (the 3rd knee bone) presents a ditch, because the back end is pointing downward. This ditch is still better seen in a view from below of the same bones (Fig. 50). The radiograph of the lower row of the bones of the right knee appears in Fig. 51. There are many cysts at the back end of the 3rd and 4th knee bones. Bone slabs from the front end to the back end of the 3rd and 4th knee bones are presented in Fig. 52. In such sections, the bones should be rectangular with well defined corners, but instead the lower back corner of the 3rd knee bone is pointing backward and downward with a big gap between the two pieces. Similar but less advanced changes occur in the 4th knee bone. In the radiographs of these slab sections (Fig. 53), a large area without radiographic density separates the lower back end of the 3rd knee bone and the main portion. Again, similar but less advanced changes occur in the 4th knee bone. Under the microscope (Fig. 54), the area without radiographic density is shown to be retained cartilage. The cartilage destined to form the

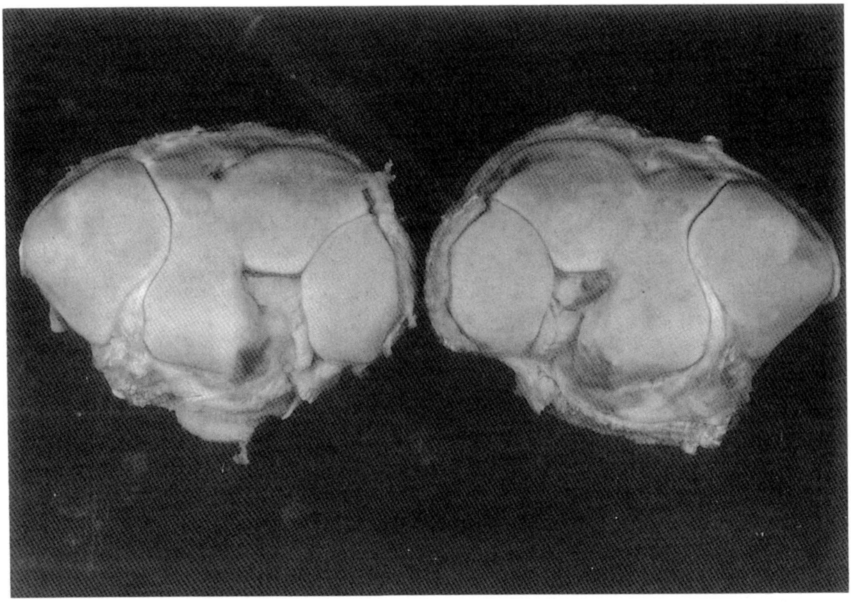

Fig. 49. The lower row of knee bones, seen from above. The left row is to the left and the bones are, from the left, 4th, 3rd and 2nd knee bones. The right bones, are from the left, 2nd, 3rd and 4th knee bones. The back side (bottom) of the 3rd knee bones shows a ditch in the cartilage.

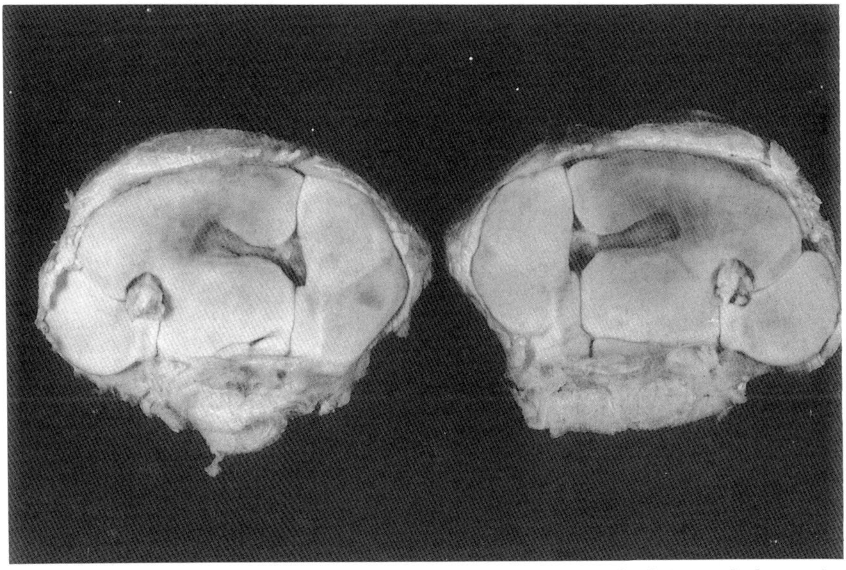

Fig. 50. The lower row of knee bones seen from below. The ditch is much deeper in the lower side. The round structure between the 4th and 3rd knee bones and between the 3rd and 2nd knee bones is normal. Note that a deep groove in the cartilage extends transversely into the 3rd carpal bones from the round structure between the 4th and 3rd knee bone in both rows.

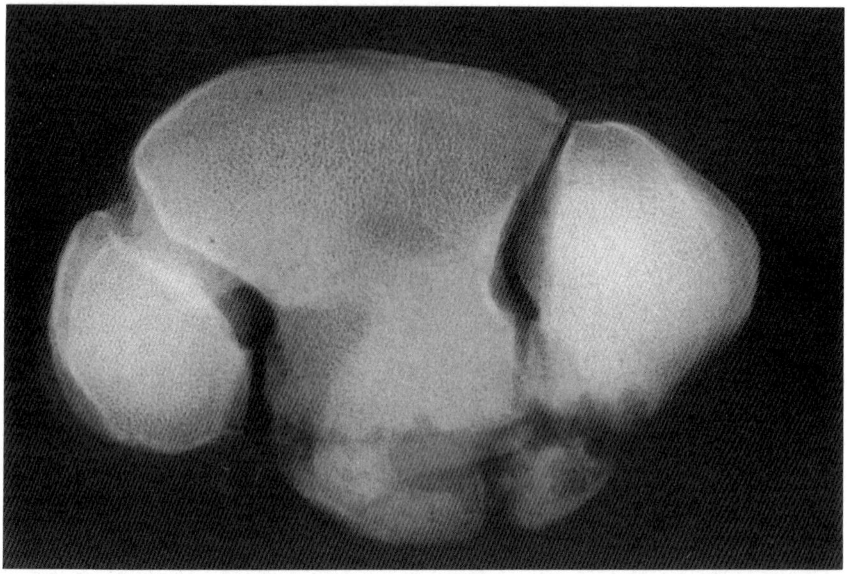

Fig. 51. Radiograph of the lower row of right knee bones; the 4th knee bone is to the right. The 3rd (middle) and 4th knee bones present several large cysts (the dark areas) at the back side.

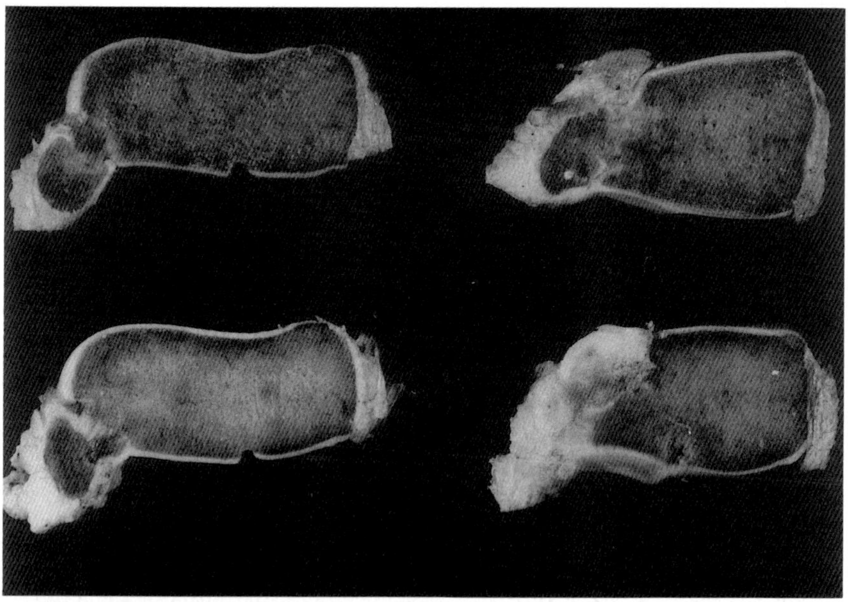

Fig. 52. Slab sections through the 3rd knee bones (left) and of the 4th knee bones (right) cut from the front end to the back end. The bones from the left knee are at top, those of the right at bottom. The lower back corner of the 3rd knee bones points backward and downward and is separated from the main bone by a large chunk of cartilage. Similar but much less pronounced changes occur in the 4th knee bones.

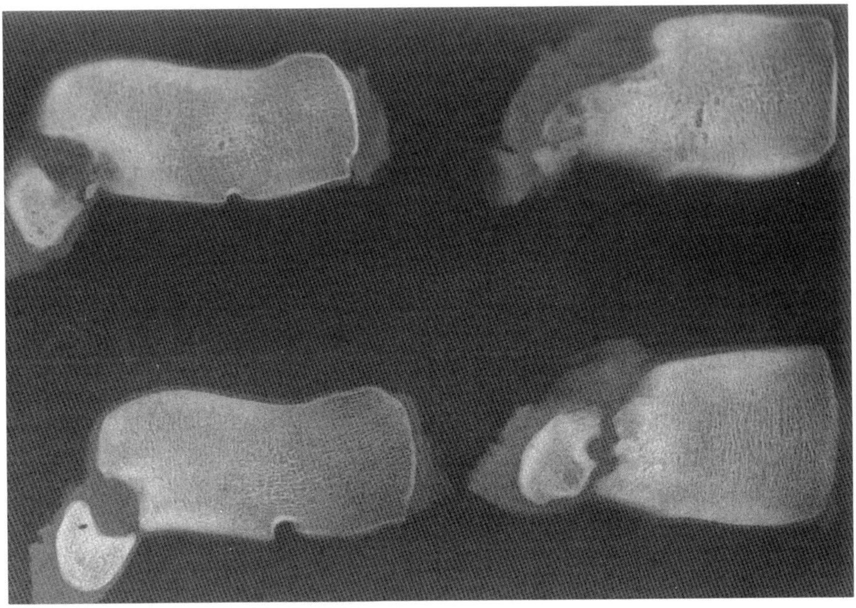

Fig. 53. Radiographs of the slab section in Fig. 52, arranged in the same way. There is a large area without radiographic density separating the lower back corner of the 3rd knee bone from the main bone. Less advanced changes occur in the 4th knee bone.

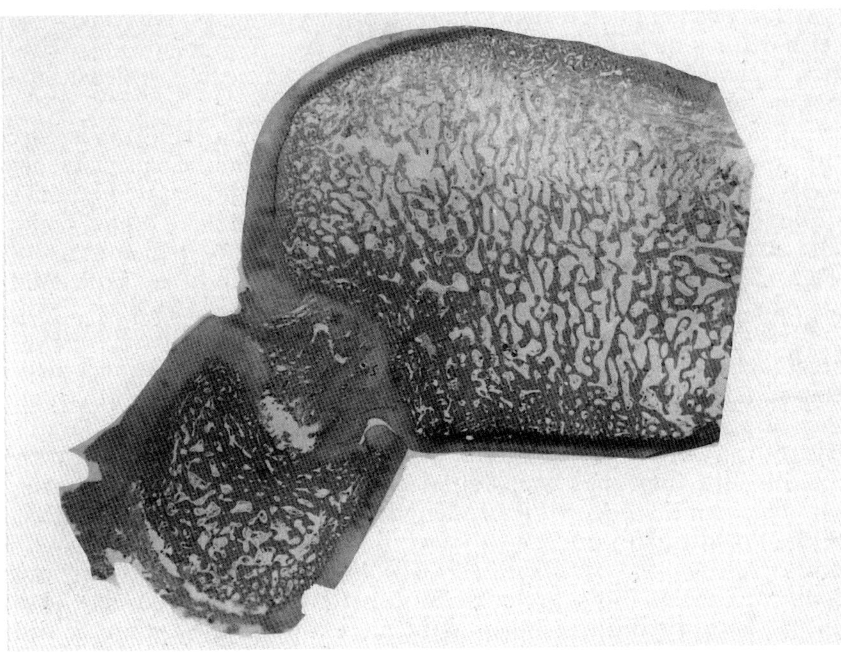

Fig. 54. Microscopic section of the lower back area of the left 3rd knee bone. The back side is to the left. There is a large chunk of cartilage between the main part of the 3rd knee bone and the big piece of bone pointing backward and downward. ×2.1.

lower back corner of the 3rd knee bone did not do its job but remained there as retained cartilage, resulting in a vastly mis-shaped 3rd knee bone.

The suspensory ligament attaches at its upper end to the lower half of the back side of the lower row of knee bone and to the most upper part of the cannon bone. It then runs downward on the back side of the cannon bone and divides at the lower ¼ of that bone; the branches embrace the sesamoid bones, move forward, and join the extensor tendon on the front side of the long pastern bone. In the case under discussion, the attachment of the suspensory ligament had been displaced downward about ½ an inch or more because of OCH in the 3rd and 4th knee bones of both limbs. The fetlock joint was, therefore, extended and the knee flexed. This is a case of OCH, of which the so-called contraction of the flexor tendon is only a secondary manifestation.

2. So-called epiphysitis

Epiphysis, as defined in Chapter III, is the region of the growth plate and of the end of the bone just above or below the plate. The word ending -itis means inflammation. The term epiphysitis thus means an inflammation of the epiphysis. As applied to the condition in horses, the term is wrong and misleading, because there is no inflammation. Another term applied to define the condition is angular deformity. The term defines the clinical appearance but it does not include any defintion of the nature of the disease, far less of its cause, but, at least, it is not an inaccurate term.

The angular deformity concerns the knee region. The long axis of the cannon bone and that of the forearm bone should normally describe a straight line. Axis is defined as "an imaginary line passing through the center of a body," in this case the middle of a long bone. The straight line is not present in Fig. 55, the knee region of an 8-week-old quarterhorse filly. The axis of the forearm bone is deviated outward (for details, see the legend of Fig. 55).

Now to the case of the 2-year-old thoroughbred filly. By microscopic examination of the forearm, we have a good idea what is happening and why it is happening. In Fig. 56, we have sections through the lower end of the left forearm. (a) of that figure shows the outer part of the left forearm cut from outside. The cartilage of the growth plate is still there but is surrounded by dense bone. Obviously, this cartilage can no longer produce lengthwise growth. In the inner part of the growth plate (b), the cartilage is well defined. There is a horizontal split in the cartilage, an OCD. Above the cartilage are tiny bone bars, which indicate that some growth is still going on. The bone above the growth plate is abundant and many of the bone bars are arranged transversely. Even with OCD within the growth plate, there

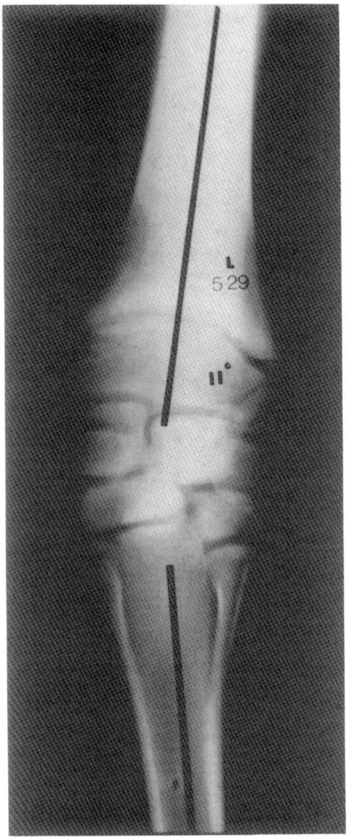

Fig. 55. Quarterhorse filly, 8-week-old. Radiograph from front of left forearm-knee-cannon bone region. The forearm bone is at top. The transverse line at the lower part of the forearm bone is the growth plates, below that is the lower epiphysis. Then come the two rows of knee bones and, at the lower part, the cannon bone. The outer splint bone is to the right of the cannon bone. Inside appears at the left, outside at the right. The long axis of the cannon bone and of the forearm bone is indicated by a black line. The axis of the forearm bone is pointing outward, at an 11-degree angle to the axis of the cannon bone. Photo courtesy of Dr. Jack Geary, New York State College of Veterinary Medicine.

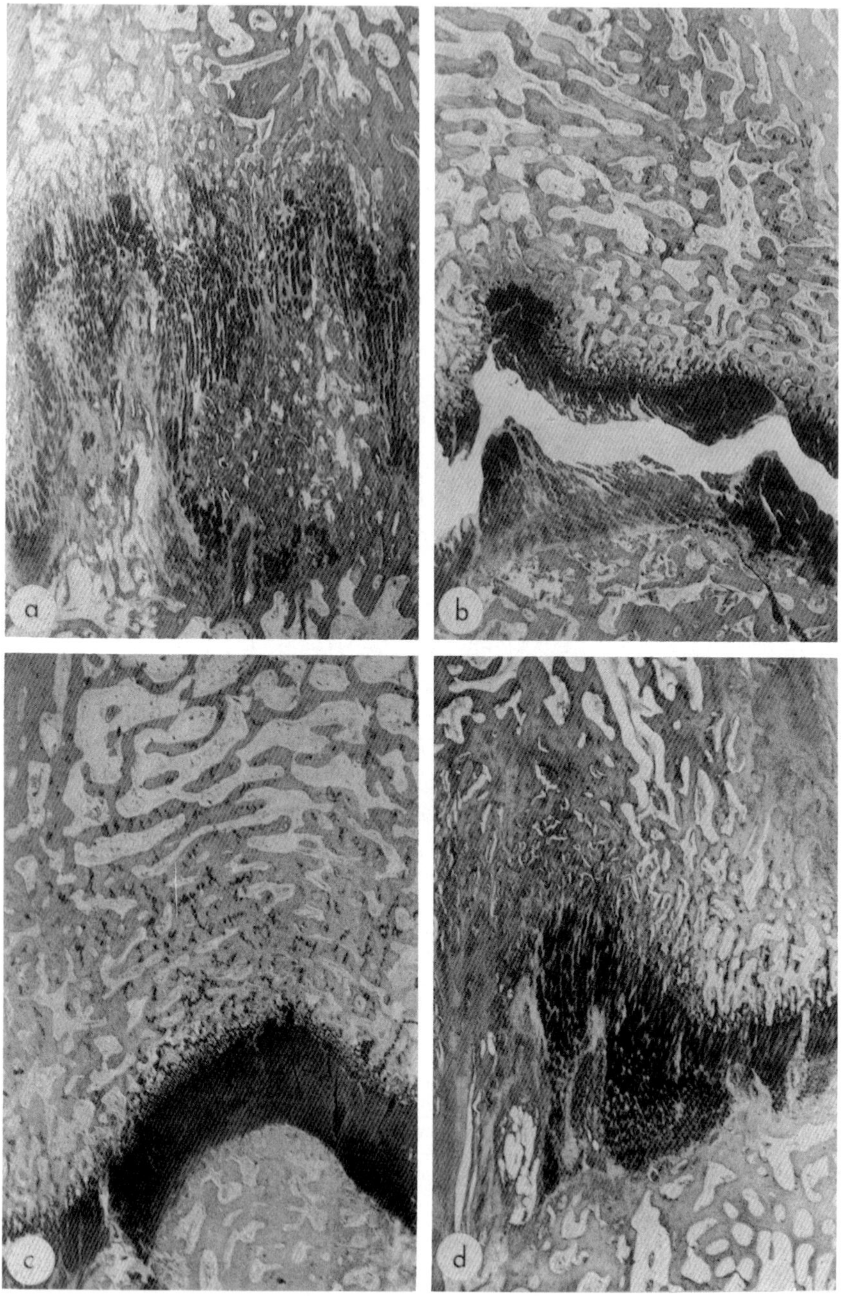
a
b
c
d

has recently been some lengthwise growth. The situation in the right limb is much the same (Figs. c and d). The inner part (c) does show some growth activity, with tiny bone bars formed by the lower end of the growth plate. The outer part (d) is much the same as the left forearm. Again, in (c), there is much too much bone in the area beyond the growth plate, and the bone bars are arranged transversely.

Even though the filly is already 2 years old, and the activity in the growth plates of the lower end of the forearm is minimal, we can reconstruct the events leading to angular deformity. The activity in the outer part of the growth plate, seen from the front, has ceased completely. In the inner part, which faces the opposite limb, there is still some activity. These late changes began long ago during active growth of the forearm. If the growth from the inner part of the plate is greater than that of the outer part, the axis of the forearm will be deviated outward. This is the very definition of "angular deformity." Based on the examination of the current case as presented in Fig. 56, this entity is another example of OCH. The following criteria of OCH are present in our case: extensive changes in the growth cartilages, including OCD and transverse trabeculation, conditions which, as discussed in Chapter IV, indicate a previous stop-and-go activity in the growth plate.

In the examination of a disease by the clinician or the pathologist, three types of diagnoses may be reached. First, there is a symptomatic diagnosis. This is based on the symptoms observed by the patient and reported to the physician. The second type of diagnosis is morphologic. The third type is an etiologic diagnosis. The etiologic diagnosis establishes the cause of a disease. Sometimes, but far from always, the symptomatic diagnosis indicates the cause. Only if an etiologic diagnosis is reached can proper treatment and, far better, prevention be applied.

In the entity under discussion, the term epiphysitis is useless for the simple reason that it is wrong. The term angular deformity is cor-

---

Fig. 56. Thoroughbred filly, 2-year-old. The microscopic sections from the lower part of the forearm are cut from outside to inside in the middle of the plane transverse from in front. a is the from the outer part of the left forearm; b is from the inner part of the left forearm; c is from the inner part of the right forearm; d is from the outer part of the right forearm. ×18.

a. The remnants of the growth plate are the dark areas, which describe wide waves rather than a straight band. The cartilage is tightly surrounded by dense bone.

b. The growth plate (black) is well defined. There is an OCD change horizontally through the plate. There is still some growth activity, as indicated by thin bone bars projecting upward from the plate. Note that there is transverse trabeculation above the plate.

c. The growth plate (black band at the bottom) does show some activity as judged by the bone bars projecting upward. There is dense bone above the plate and pronounced transverse trabeculation.

d. The situation here is much the same as in a. The growth plate is surrounded by dense bone. Growth has ceased.

rect as a symptomatic diagnosis, but it tells nothing about the nature of the disease. By establishing OCH as the morphologic basis of angular deformity, we have gone one step further, but the cause of the disease has not thereby been defined. Surgical correction only relieves the clinical signs. It does not change the underlying disease.

3. More OCH

A 2-year-old thoroughbred gelding was donated because of severe lameness, diagnosed by clinical radiographs as originating in the right stifle. The horse never trained, never raced.

The next seven illustrations are from this horse. Fig. 57 shows a radiograph of the *left* stifle region (in which no clinical signs appeared). Everything is normal by radiographic examination. Note especially the height of the spine of the tibia, the part of the tibia that projects upward into the area between the lower joint bones (the condyles) of the thigh bone.

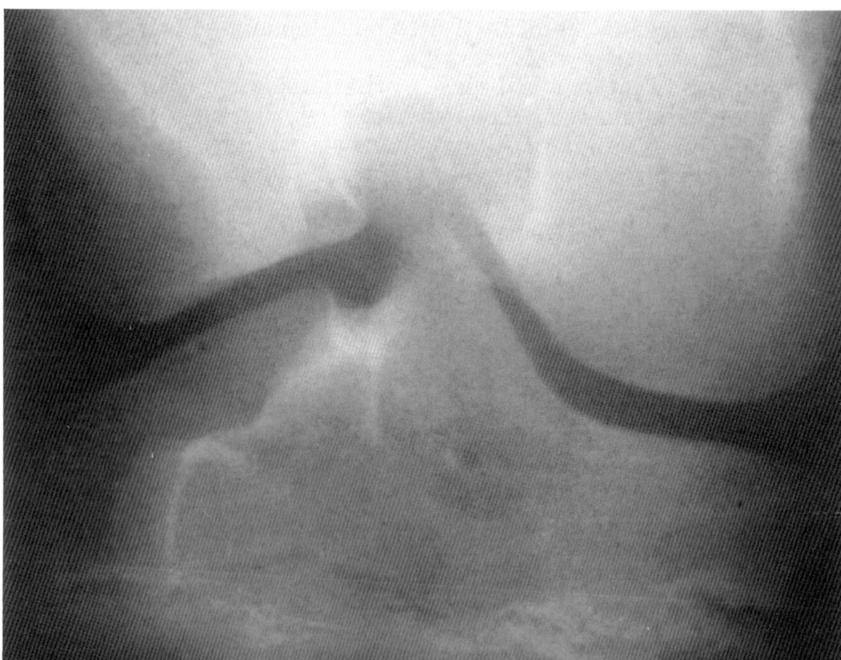

Fig. 57. Thoroughbred gelding, 2-year-old. Clinical radiograph of the *left* stifle region exposed from behind. At the top is the lower end of the thigh bone, and below is the upper end of the tibia. Outside is to the left. The large inner condyle of the thigh bone (upper right) plays against the concave inner upper end of the tibia. The spine of the tibia projects high up into the area between the condyles of the thigh bone.

Now we compare the left stifle to the right one, where we find the reason for the lameness. The spine is flattened because of a large cyst (Fig. 58) where you should normally find the spine of the tibia. The joint surface of the inner upper part, against which the large inner condyle of the thigh bone plays, is flat, not concave.

The cyst demonstrated by radiography (Fig. 58) is shown in a slab section from outside to inside of the upper end of the tibia in Fig. 59. In this plane, the inner part of the joint does not show the normal concavity. A radiograph (Fig. 60) of this slab section, about ¼ inch thick, reveals that the cyst is much larger than suggested by inspection of the surface (Fig. 59). The spine is absent in the radiograph (Fig. 60).

The changes in the middle region of the slab section are not restricted to the spine. In a slab section, parallel but much further back, we see the same changes (Fig. 61). They now appear beneath the joint cartilage of the inner joint area of the upper end of the tibia. In the same picture, the growth plate shows very advanced irregularities.

The changes depicted in Figs. 57-61 show that we are dealing with OCH, with catastrophic results in the upper end of the right tibia. The next two pictures are presented to show that the changes

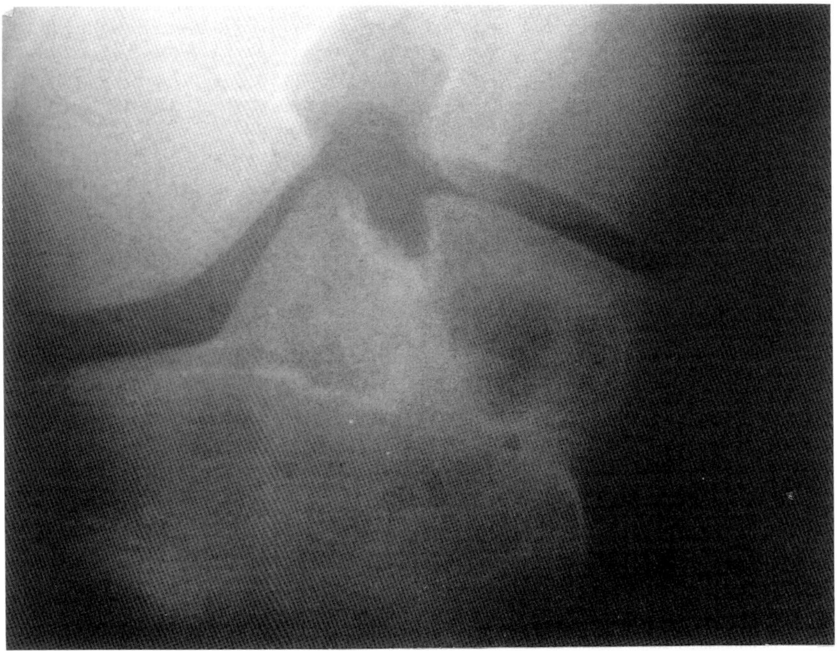

Fig. 58. Clinical radiograph of the *right* stifle area arranged as in Fig. 57. Outside is to the right. The spine is flattened because of a large cyst at the top. The contour of the inner upper end of the tibia is not as regular as that on the left side in Fig. 57.

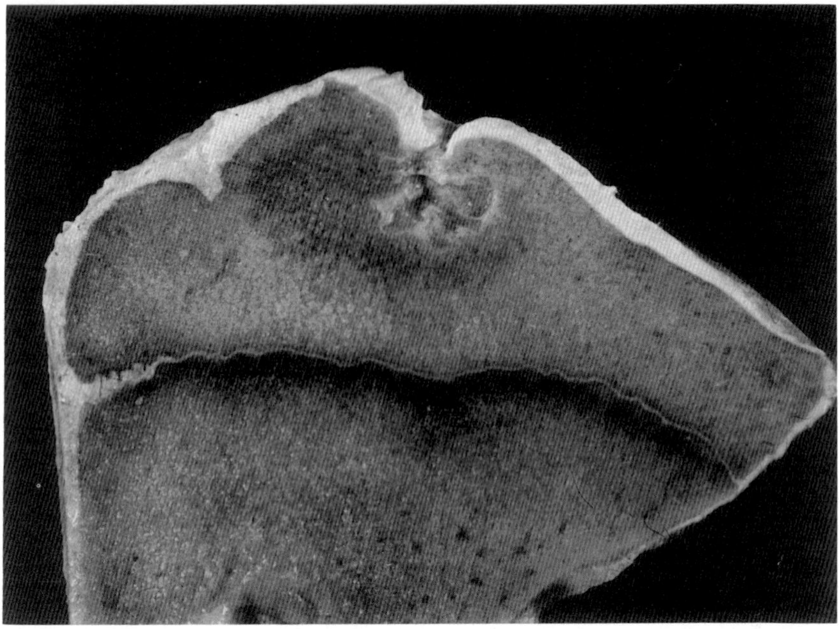

Fig. 59. Slab section through the upper end of the right tibia cut from outside (left) to inside. There is a large cyst beneath the area that should have been the spine. In this plane, the inner part surface does not show the normal concavity. Note that joint cartilage of the outer surface projects into the bone.

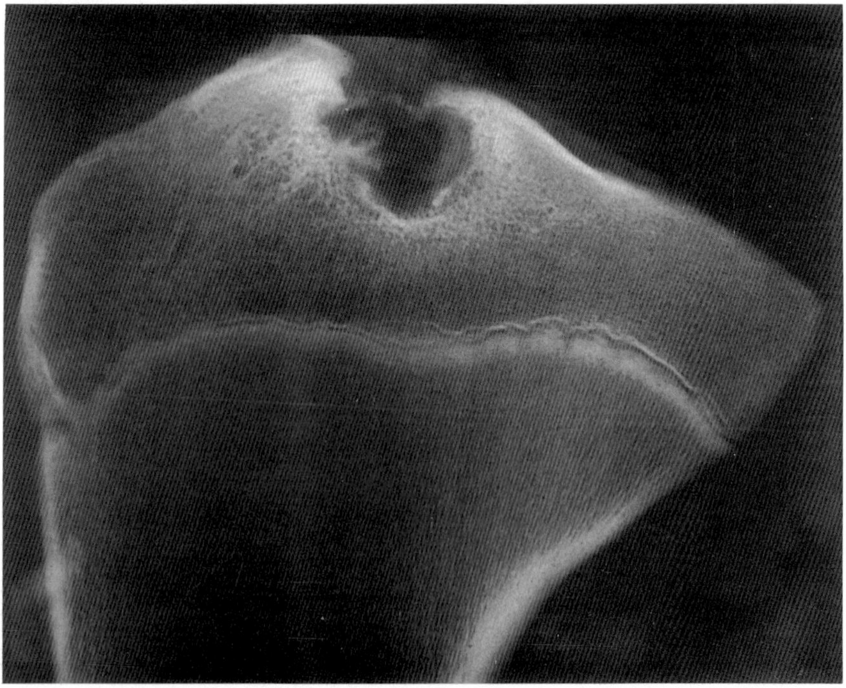

Fig. 60. In the radiograph of the ¼-inch thick slab section in Fig. 59, the extent of the cyst is much greater. The spine is absent.

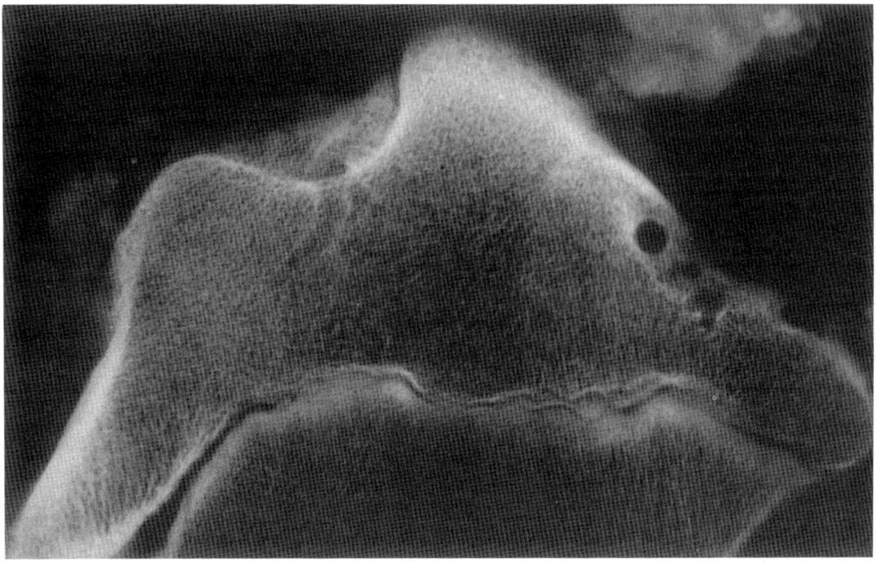

Fig. 61. Radiograph of a slab section parallel but further back from that of Fig. 60. There are several cysts beneath the joint cartilage of the inner upper end. Note also the irregular appearance of the growth plate.

are generalized. We see in Fig. 62 a radiograph of the right knee, exposed from the side. In the outer bone of the upper row (the ulnar knee bone) is a large "hole." When sliced and examined under the microscope, this "cyst" was shown to be a large area of retained cartilage.

As further evidence of the generalized nature of OCH, we see in Fig. 63 the lower end of the right arm bone. There are many longitudinal and deep grooves in the joint cartilage. The grooves were formed because detached pieces of cartilage acted as grinding material. The grooves, thus, represent an event caused by OCH, not, as commonly stated, a result of wear and tear.

We now have before us yet another case of OCH. Because of the failure to develop a spine of the right tibia, the thigh bone slipped toward the outer side and created pressure on the joint capsule, resulting in pain and lameness. The horse never took a normal step in his short life, and could not be trained, let alone race.

REFERENCE

1. Jeffcott, L.B., P.D. Rossdale, J. Freestone, C.J. Frank and P.F. Towers-Clark. 1982. An assessment of wastage in thoroughbred racing from conception to 4 years of age. Equine vet. J. *14:*185-198.

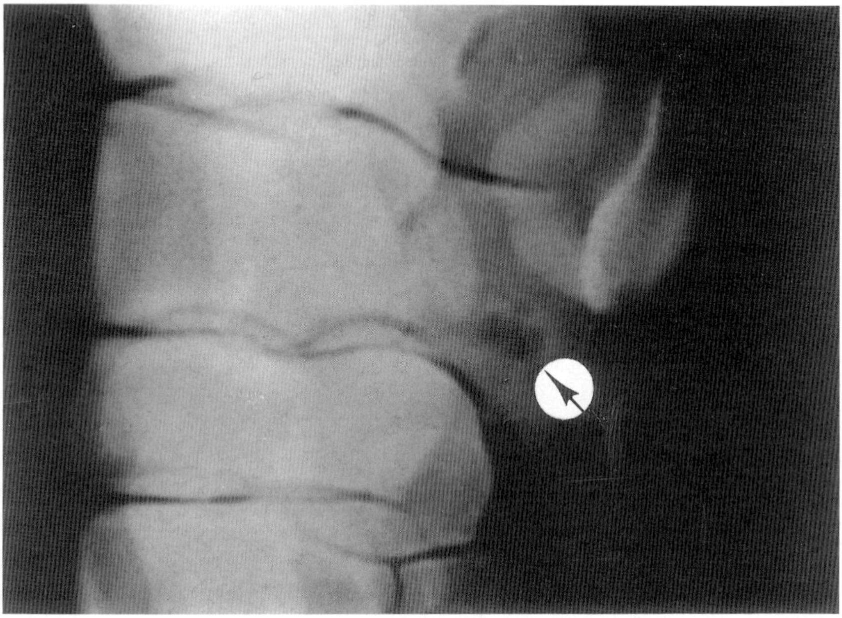

Fig. 62. Radiograph of the right knee seen from the side. In front of the arrow is a large cyst in the outer bone of the upper row of knee bones (ulnar knee bone).

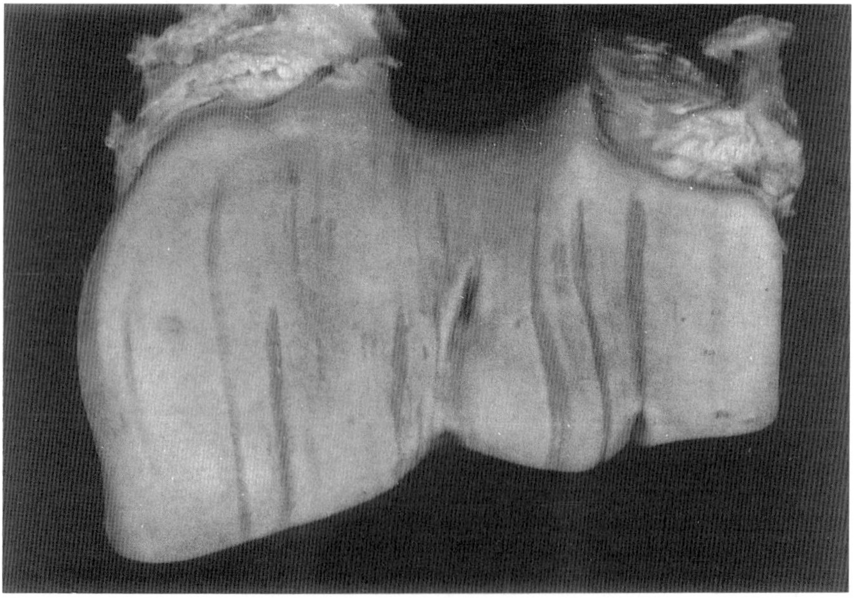

Fig. 63. Lower end of the *right* arm bone. There are numerous deep grooves in the joint cartilage.

VI. TRACK CONDITION AND RACING INJURIES IN THOROUGHBRED HORSES

Fractures are broadly classified as either traumatic or pathologic. Traumatic means that a violent external force acts on the bone or bones to cause the fracture. Pathologic means that the fracture occurred because of a disease of the bone or bones.

Fractured bones in race horses are conventionally and conveniently considered traumatic and caused by bad track condition. No one has offered an explanation of bad track conditions but the term is used nonetheless. What we need here are numbers. We have published (1) a study entitled "Track condition and racing injuries in thoroughbred horses". The following information is extracted from that report.

The records on racing injuries by the Chief Examining Veterinarian of the New York Racing Association (NYRA) tracks from February 1, 1983, through mid-October, 1985, were analyzed. NYRA operates three tracks: Aqueduct, Jamaica, NY; Belmont Park, Elmont, NY; and Saratoga, Saratoga Springs, NY.

Aqueduct, with racing from November to April, has two dirt tracks, main and inner and one turf course. The circumference of the dirt tracks are 1⅛ mile and 1 mile, respectively. The turf track circumference is 7 furlongs, 43 feet.

Belmont Park, with racing from April to November with the exception of August, has one dirt track with a circumference of 1½ mile. The Widener or main turf track is 1 5/16 mile, 27 feet and the inner turf track is 1 3/16 mile, 103 feet.

Saratoga, with racing in August, has one dirt track which measures 1⅛ mile. The main turf track is 1 mile, 98 feet, and the inner turf track is 7 furlongs, 304 feet.

During the period stated above, there were 68,397 starts at the NYRA tracks.

Dirt track conditions are classified as Fast, Good, Muddy, and Sloppy. Turf track conditions are classified as Firm, Good, Soft, and Yielding.

Racing injuries were recorded as fracture injuries (FI) and other injuries (OI). OI concern soft tissues and include nose bleeding, muscle soreness, joint soreness, tendon and ligament injuries, bucked shins, contusions and lacerations, etc. The sum of FI and OI is referred to as all injuries (AI).

In Table 1 is an analysis of injuries recorded during races on various track conditions. There were no differences in injuries no matter what the track condition.

Table 1. Dirt track condition and racing injuries. FI = fracture injuries, OI = other injuries, AI = all injuries

Track	Total	Fast	Good	Muddy	Sloppy
Starts	57970	47336	3456	3063	4015
FI	123	97	5	10	11
OI	314	265	16	13	20
AI	437	362	21	23	31

No significant differences

Table 2 is a comparison of racing injuries on the three NYRA tracks. Fracture injuries were higher at Saratoga than at Aqueduct. We have no explanation for this. Soft tissue injuries were the same, but because of higher fracture incidence at Saratoga, the AI were also higher.

Table 2. Racing injuries on dirt tracks

Track	Aqueduct		Belmont	Saratoga
	Main	Inner		
Starts	15067	19027	20148	3728
FI	23	38	51	11
OI	81	116	98	19
AI	104	154	149	30

FI: Saratoga > Aqueduct

On turf tracks (Table 3), the track condition did not influence the incidence of racing injuries at all, and there were no differences in the number of injuries on the different NYRA tracks (Table 4).

Table 3. Turf track condition and racing injuries

Track	Total	Firm	Good	Soft	Yielding
Starts	10427	7714	1822	492	399
FI	11	9	1	1	0
OI	49	39	6	3	1
AI	60	48	7	4	1

No significant differences

Table 4. Racing injuries on turf tracks

Track	Aqueduct	Belmont		Saratoga	
		Main	Inner	Main	Inner
Starts	894	4222	3402	1181	728
FI	1	7	3	0	0
OI	3	16	22	2	6
AI	4	23	25	2	6

No significant differences

When we compare the fracture incidence on dirt tracks to that on turf track, we find (Table 5) that the incidence is higher on dirt tracks. Fig. 64 shows the OI to FI ratio with increasing age. In 2-year-olds,

Table 5. Racing injuries on dirt and turf tracks

Track	Dirt	Turf
Starts	57970	10427
FI	123	11
OI	314	49
AI	437	60

FI: Dirt > turf

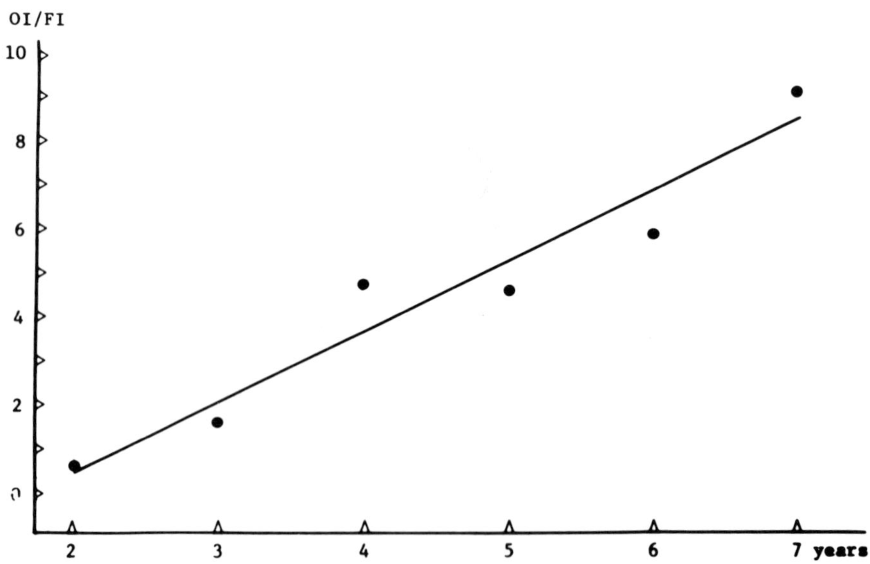

Fig. 64. On the vertical axis to the left is the ratio between other injuries (OI) and fracture injuries (FI); on the horizontal axis is the age of horses.

At 2 years of age, the ratio is less than one, which means that there are more fractures than soft tissue (other) injuries. With increasing age, the ratio becomes higher, which means that fractures are becoming fewer and soft tissue injuries more frequent.

the ratio is less than one and then increases with increasing age. In other words, fractures concern mainly young horses. Table 6 shows that the 2-year-olds account for 14% of all starts on dirt tracks but only for 7 percent on turf tracks. Dirt track races start at least 3

Table 6. Starts by 2-year-olds on dirt and turf tracks

	Dirt		Turf	
All ages	21836		3533	
2-year-olds	3072	(14 percent)	246	(7 percent)

Dirt > turf

months earlier than do turf races. The dirt track horses are, thus, 3 months younger when first racing than the turf track horses. All these facts seem to explain the higher incidence of FI on dirt tracks and to indicate that there is no difference in FI on dirt and turf tracks.

The pole position in races in which FI occurred were recorded in 53 cases which are plotted in Fig. 65. FI occurred at the start, at the end, and anywhere in between.

Only for 6 furlong races were there enough data to allow for statistical analysis. This analysis shows that there are, statistically, similar incidences of fractures during the first and second half of the race. In other words, distance run does not influence the incidence of fractures.

The seasonal distribution of FI and AI is accounted for in Table 7. There is, by statistical analysis, no seasonal influence. For the four warmest months, June through September, the average rank score for FI is 4, exactly the same as for the three coldest months, December through February. The average rank scores for OI for the same periods are similar (5.75 and 6.33, respectively).

The influence of cold temperatures on FI and OI were recorded from data on the inner dirt track of Aqueduct (Table 8). Temperatures from 10° Fahrenheit to more than 50° Fahrenheit did not significantly affect the incidence of FI and OI.

The conclusion of analyses of racing injuries during 68,397 starts at NYRA tracks is that track condition, kind of track, length of races, and environmental conditions are not of decisive importance on the incidence of racing injuries.

There were 134 FI and 363 OI during 68,397 starts, which is 0.2 percent FI and 0.53 percent OI. These figures, however, are deceptively low. If we assume that a horse starts 10 times a year, then the

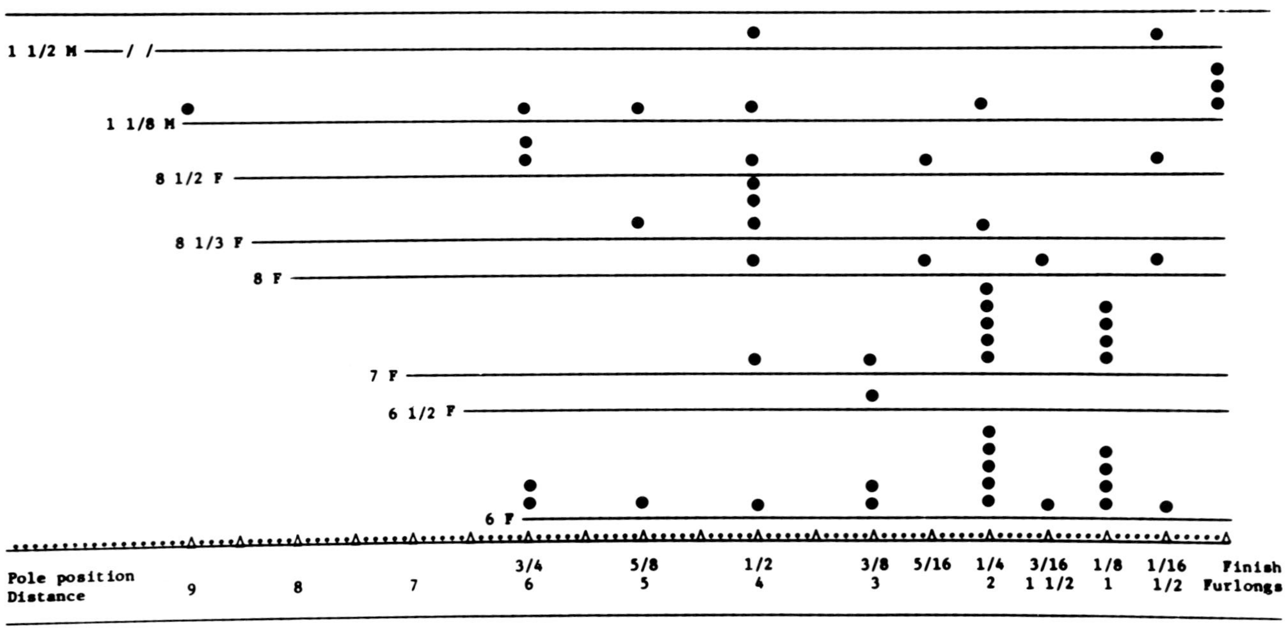

Fig. 65. Each black dot indicates the location where a fracture occurred. On the bottom line, the fractures in 6-furlong races are plotted. Then, going upward we have 6½-furlong races, 7-furlong races, an so on up to 1½ mile races. Fractures can occur at the start, at the finish, and anywhere in between.

Table 7. Monthly distribution of FI and OI

Month	Starts	FI	FI/1000 starts	OI	OI/1000 starts	FI rank	OI rank
January	4315	11	2.55	20	4.63	3	8
February	5937	11	1.85	41	6.91	7	2
March	6463	7	1.08	47	7.27	11	1
April	6176	11	1.78	32	5.18	8	7
May	6175	9	1.46	23	3.72	9	11
June	6423	20	3.11	41	6.38	1	3
July	6270	15	2.39	33	5.26	4	6
August	6283	12	1.91	36	5.73	6	4
September	6089	13	2.15	27	4.43	5	10
October	5648	8	1.42	20	3.54	10	12
November	4220	4	0.95	23	5.45	12	5
December	4398	13	2.96	20	4.55	2	9

No significant differences

Table 8. Influence of air temperature (Fahrenheit) on FI and OI

Temp. F	Starts	FI	FI/1000 starts	OI	OI/1000 starts	FI rank	OI rank
10-20	799	1	1.25	4	5.01	5	5
21-30	3688	11	2.98	20	5.42	2	3
31-40	6372	9	1.41	32	5.02	4	4
41-50	6710	12	1.79	49	7.30	3	2
>50	1458	5	3.43	11	7.54	1	1

No significant differences

risk figures for FI and OI would be 10 times as great. Injuries are more common during training than during racing. This, of course, increases still more the total incidence of FI and OI for horses that made it to training and racing.

There are no comparable analyses from other tracks. We will, therefore, point out that what has been stated in this chapter concerns NYRA tracks only and only for the period listed. Whether our findings are applicable to other thoroughbred race tracks in the US and elsewhere will depend on future statistical analyses from other tracks. We stand by our data even though they may not always agree with experience.

We should further point out that our analyses concern only thoroughbred flat races. We have no data on thoroughbred steeplechase races and no data from standardbred racing.

REFERENCE

1. Hill, T., D. Carmichael, G. Maylin and L. Krook. 1986. Track condition and racing injuries in thoroughbred horses. Cornell Vet., *76:*361-379.

VII. FRACTURES IN THOROUGHBRED RACE HORSES

1. Traumatic or pathologic fractures?

We have studied 53 fracture cases occurring during races at Finger Lakes Race Track, Canadaigua, NY and at NYRA tracks. The horses were destroyed at the track, trucked to New York State College of Veterinary Medicine, and examined on the same or the next day.

In all but 2 cases, a disease was diagnosed in bones or tendons. The fractures are, thus, pathologic. Failure to show a disease in 2 cases may well be because of inadequate sampling for examination. Though gross diagnosis of a fracture is very simple, it rarely establishes the cause of the fracture. The same goes for radiologic examination. Microscopic examination is absolutely necessary and, for that reason, we will present numerous microscopic pictures to show the nature of the disease underlying fractures.

Three different types of diseases were found to cause fractures:

A. Osteochondrosis;

B. Chondro-osteo-necrosis; and

C. Tendon degeneration.

A. Osteochondrosis (OCH) is defined as a failure of cartilage to convert into bone. Chapter III, "DEVELOPMENT OF BONES" served as a basis for the understanding of OCH which was described and illustrated in Chapter IV. There is more to come on OCH in this chapter.

B. Chondro-osteo-necrosis. This tongue-twister, for which there is no popular term, is called CON for short. The term CON means death of cartilage and bone beginning in the cartilage.

First, take another look at Fig. 23 in Chapter III. You see that the joint cartilage has plenty of cells and that the cartilage is stained dark. Now we shall compare this normal picture to that of CON. The horse was a 7-year-old thoroughbred gelding, which had had bad knees for several years. He won 5 races in 1983 and 2 in 1984 but ran poorly on July 4, 1984. In 1983, he was injected "about 6 times" with corticosteroids into the left knee. Because of his poor performance, the horse was donated to our study program.

Fig. 66 shows a microscopic field of the front end of the left third knee bone (the largest bone of the lower row of knee bones). The carti-

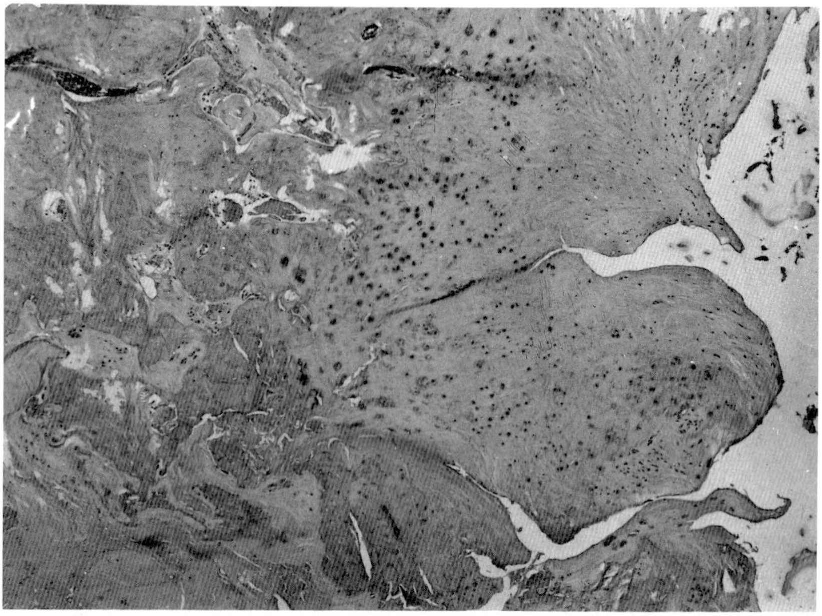

Fig. 66. Thoroughbred 7-year-old gelding which was injected 6 times during the last year with corticosteroids into the left knee. The picture shows the front end (right) of the left third knee bone. The surface of the cartilage shows a very irregular contour with deep cracks. Cells are few, and the cartilage is pale. ×40.

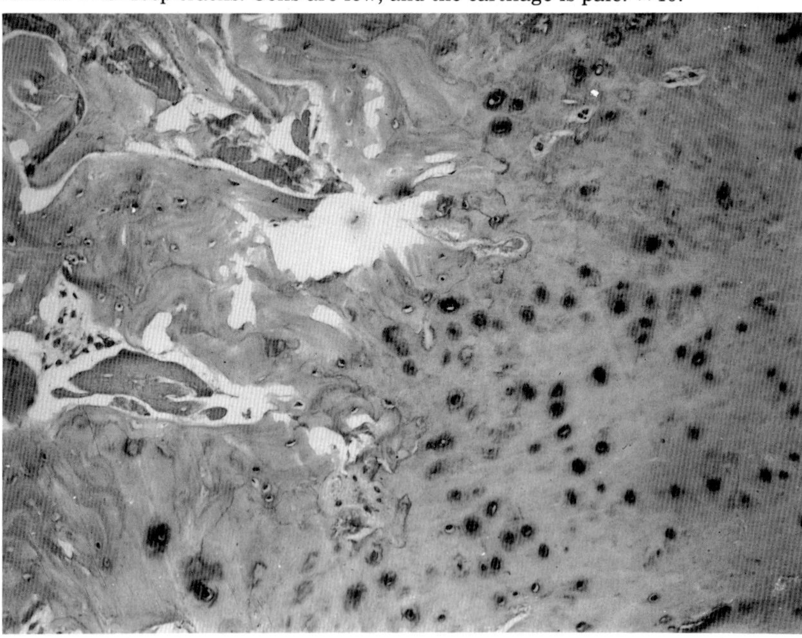

Fig. 67. Higher magnification of the field in Fig. 66. The inner part of the cartilage shows necrosis, disintegration of cells, and of the underlying bone. ×120.

lage surface is very irregular with deep cracks. Cells are few, and the cartilage is pale. Under higher microscopic magnification (Fig. 67) it becomes clear that the cartilage cells facing the underlying bone are dead and that the cartilage is falling apart, as is the underlying bone. This vast destruction of cartilage and bone can result in the picture shown in Fig. 68. We see here the upper row of the left knee seen from

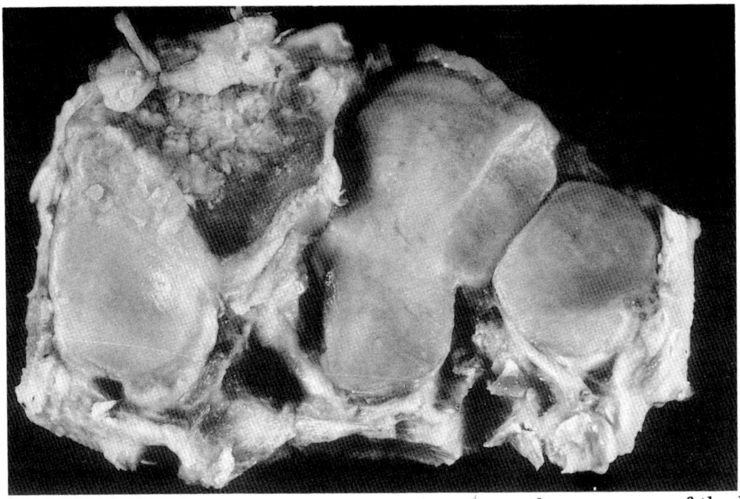

Fig. 68. Same horse as in Fig. 66. The picture shows the upper row of the left knee bones, seen from below. In the largest bone to the left (the radial knee bone) is a huge area devoid of cartilage, with the underlying bone exposed.

below. The inner knee bone (radial knee bone) presents a large area without cartilage cover and exposure of dead bone. No wonder the horse did not run well, with left knee bones so badly damaged by the injection of corticosteroids. The right knee bones were normal by gross examination.

C. Tendon degeneration

A tendon is a connective tissue cord in which muscle fibers end; a tendon, attaches to a bone or bones. In the tendon tissue, the only cells are the fibroblasts, the cells forming the fibers. As a tendon is first formed during fetal life, the fibroblasts dominate, but as collagen is produced, the fibroblasts become relatively few, with the collagen fibers dominating the microscopic field.

In the relaxed state, the collagen fibers are arranged in waves as illustrated in Fig. 69. These waves allow for stretching during loading of the tendon. Ligaments are principally the same as tendons.

The first sign of tendon degeneration is a swelling and even breaking up of the collagen. Fibers so damaged are prone to calcification, that is, deposition of calcium salts (Fig. 70). Here we see these calcium salts deposited as a fine dust. The deposits can also appear as

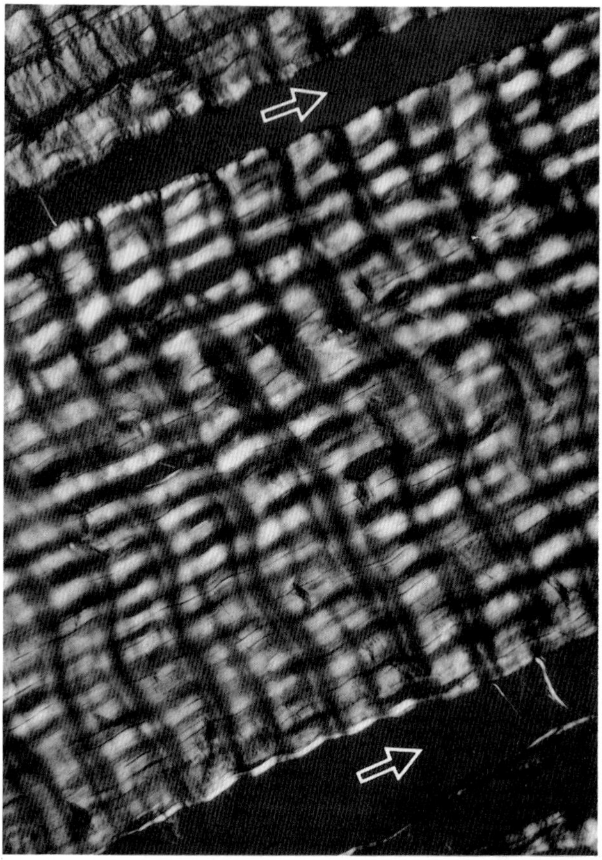

Fig. 69. Thoroughbred 4-year-old gelding that fractured the left carpus. The picture shows the deep flexor tendon of the left front limb. Polarized light exposure shows the waviness of the collagen in a *normal* tendon. The arrows indicate the lengthwise direction of the tendon. $\times 120$.

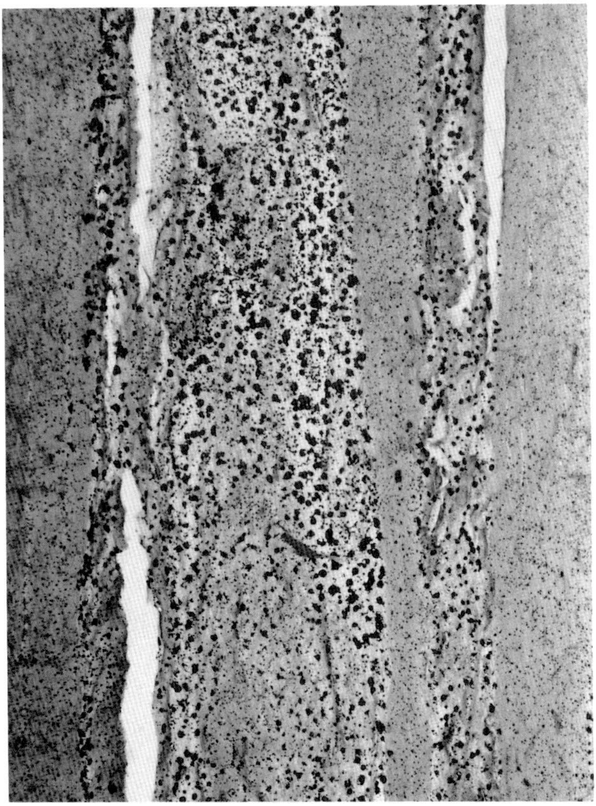

Fig. 70. A 7-year-old thoroughbred gelding which fractured both right sesamoid bones. The picture shows the deep flexor tendon of the right front limb. The fibers in the center are degenerate and are breaking up. The black spots in these fibers are calcium salts, as revealed by a specific stain called von Kossa. ×180.

thick, dense strands within the tendon (Fig. 71) or in many patches in the tendon (Fig. 72). The calcification may be so severe as to show up in the radiograph of the flexor tendons (Fig. 73).

The initial damage to the tendon tissue triggers the formation of scar tissue, which may replace large areas of degenerate tendon tissue

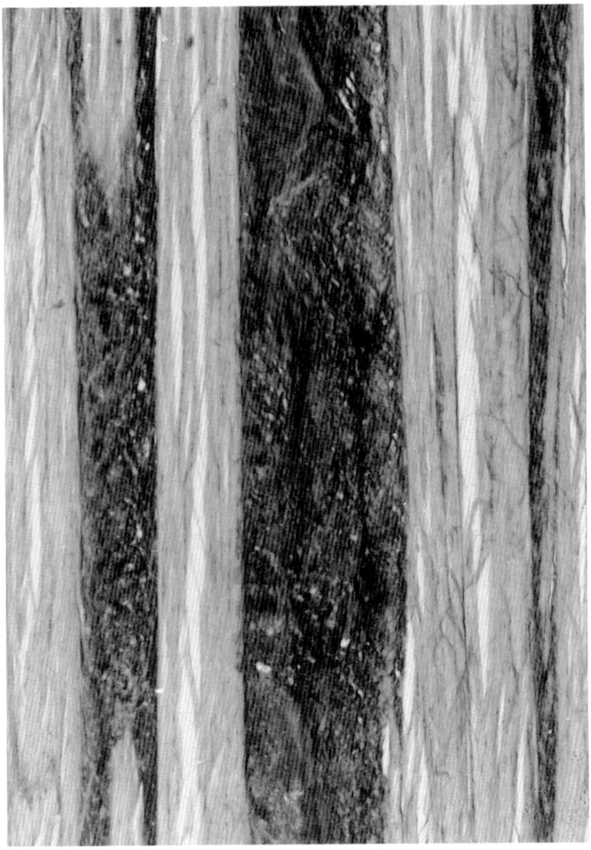

Fig. 71. A 4-year-old thoroughbred filly that fractured the left front cannon bone. The picture shows the left front deep flexor tendon. The black strands represent heavy deposits of calcium salts obscuring the dead fibers. ×45.

(Fig. 74). With regular microscopic light the difference between undamaged tendon tissue and scar tissue is not striking. When the same field is exposed with polarized light (Fig. 75), however, the difference does become striking. The normal tendon tissue absorbs polarized light, but the scar tissue does not.

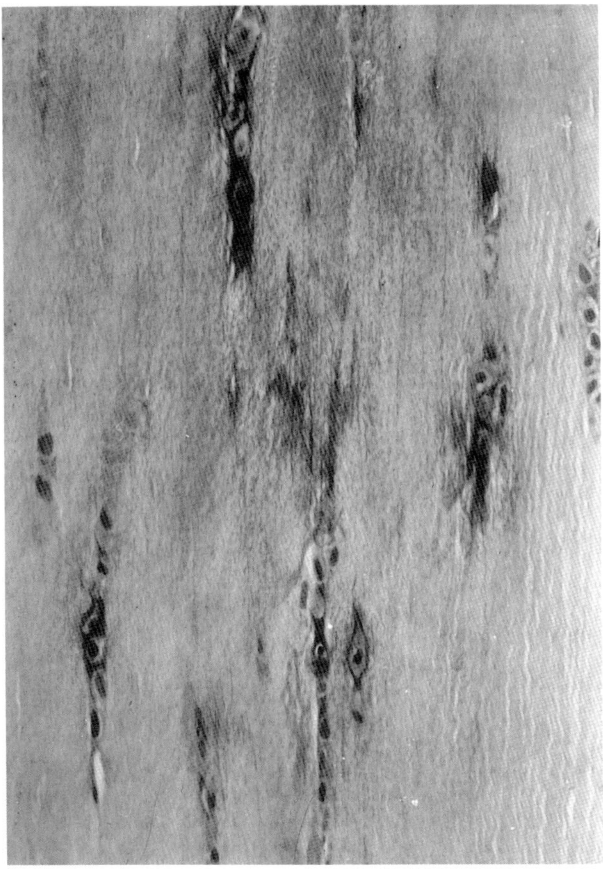

Fig. 72. A 3-year-old thoroughbred gelding that fractured the left front limb sesamoid bones. The picture shows the inner branch of the suspensory ligament. There are numerous large patches of calcium salt deposits (black areas). ×30.

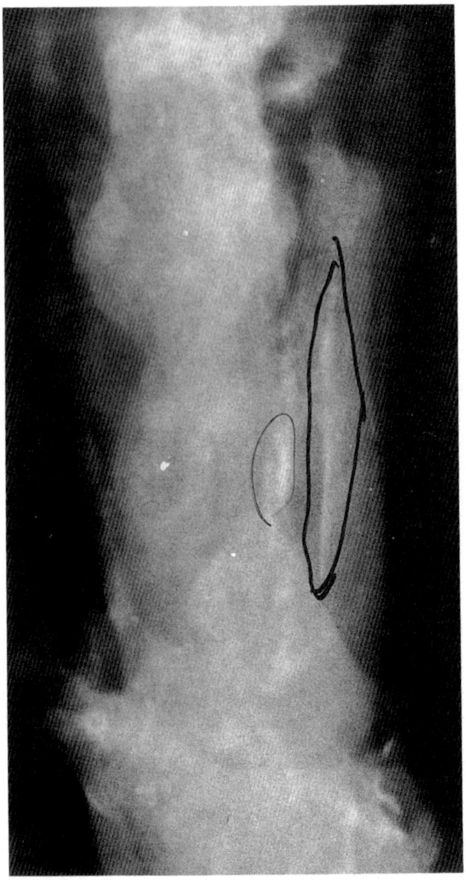

Fig. 73. A 5-year-old thoroughbred stallion that fractured the left front limb sesamoid bones. The picture shows a radiograph of the flexor tendons dessected free from the cannon bone. There are large areas of calcium deposits within the ink marks.

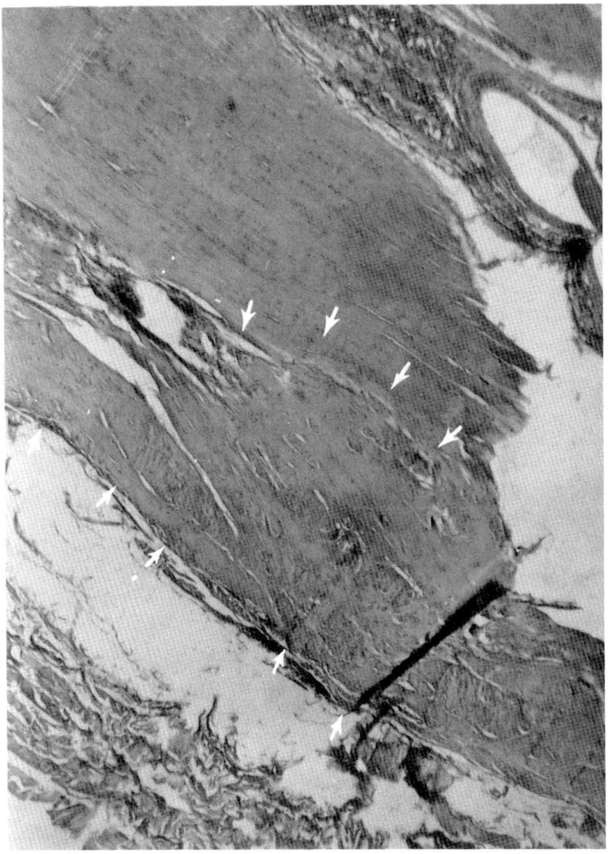

Fig. 74. This 5-year-old thoroughbred gelding fractured the left front limb cannon-bone. The picture shows the left front superficial flexor tendon. The area within the arrows consists of scar tissue with admixture of a few cartilage cells (darker area in the center). The dark area at the lower left corner represents calcium salt deposits. $\times 40$.

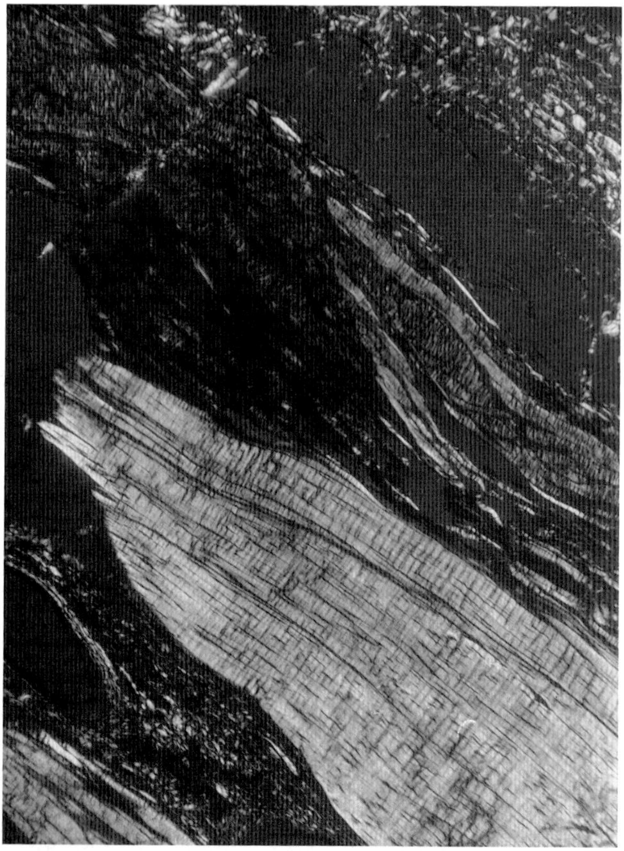

Fig. 75. Same field as in Fig. 74 exposed with polarized light. The tendon coming in from the lower right and projecting upward to the left absorbs polarized light; the scar tissue at upper middle does not.

The scar tissue sometimes shows infiltration of fat cells, which cannot fulfill any of the normal functions of tendon tissue. This is illustrated in Fig. 76. The loss of tendon tissue in this section is shown by polarized light exposure of the same field in Fig. 77.

Remarkable changes can occur in the scar tissue that replaces the tendon tissue. In Fig. 78 is a section of the deep flexor tendon of the left front limb of a 3-year-old thoroughbred gelding that fractured the left sesamoid bones during a race. There are many and extensive black areas within the scar tissue, which are bone tissue. Under higher microscopic magnification, the bone-forming cells are easily recognized (Fig. 79). The vast destruction of tendon tissue is shown, under polarized light exposure, in Fig. 80. Only a few small fragments of tendon tissue persist.

The scar tissue cells may also convert into cartilage-forming cells. This is shown in Fig. 81, a section of the deep flexor tendon of the right hind limb of a 5-year-old thoroughbred stallion that fractured the right hind coffin bone. In addition to tendon degeneration and mineral deposits, the picture shows numerous cartilage-forming cells.

A tendon or a ligament that shows degeneration, with or without mineral deposits, scar tissue, and bone and cartilage formation, has lost its normal elasticity. It can no longer respond by stretching and relaxation during movement of the limb. The stiff and unyielding tendon or ligament will, therefore, transmit abnormal mechanical forces to the bones, especially to the cannon bone, the sesamoid bones, the pastern bones, and the coffin bone. Even if these bones do not present any changes to explain the fracture, the fracture should nonetheless be considered pathological if a tendon or a ligament is damaged as described above. The bone under examination should be considered as a functional unit which includes the bone itself *with* its tendons, ligament, and joint capsule.

The cause of tendon degeneration in our material is not definitely known, but the microscopic changes are highly suggestive of the effects of corticosteroid injection; we will enlarge on this subject in the next chapter.

We will now present two pictures of tendon damage resulting from another steroid, namely vitamin D_3. The pictures are from the deep flexor tendon of a front limb of a 2-year-old thoroughbred colt. The colt was fed an estimated 400 times the recommended level of vitamin D_3. In Fig. 82 there are extensive areas of mineral deposits which occur in degenerate collagen fibers (Fig. 82a and b). In Fig. 82c, blood vessels with accompanying scar tissue cells are heading toward an area of mineral deposit. The scar tissue partially removes and replaces the degenerate and mineralized tissue (Fig. 82d). In this scar tissue is a pronounced transformation of cells into cartilage-forming cells (Figs. 83a and b). The cartilage cells sometimes mimic the arrangement of a growth plate (Fig. 83c) which, indeed, has the ability to produce bone tissue (Fig. 83d). Because of these changes in the tendons, the colt was severely lame and never made it to training.

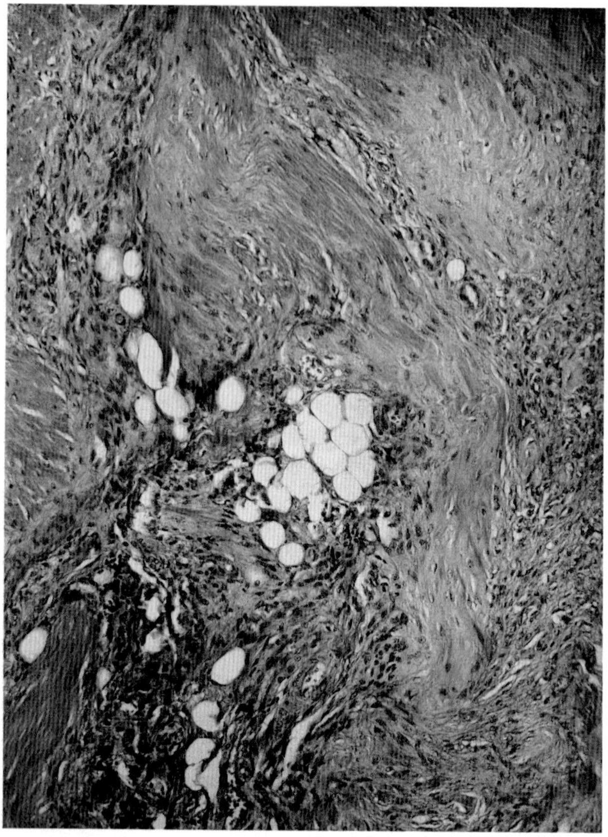

Fig. 76. This 3-year-old thoroughbred gelding fractured both sesamoid bones of the left front limb. The picture shows the outer branch of the suspensory ligament of the left front limb. There is only a little tendon tissue left, which appears at the upper left and continues down to the right. The rest of the field is occupied by scar tissue in which there are many fat cells. ×120.

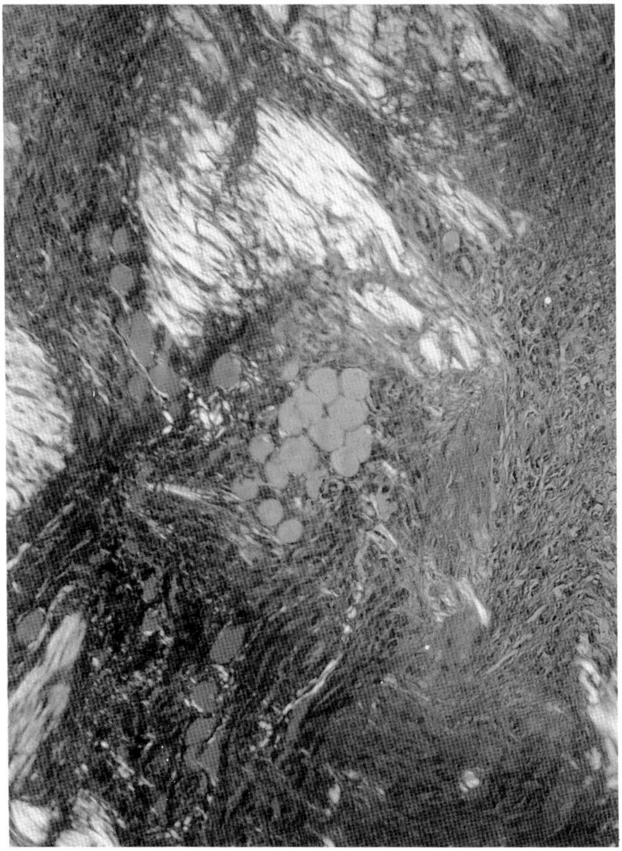

Fig. 77. Same field as in Fig. 76 exposed with polarized light. The bright areas are tendon tissue of which there is not much left. The replacing scar tissue does not absorb polarized light. The large, empty ballooned cells are fat cells.

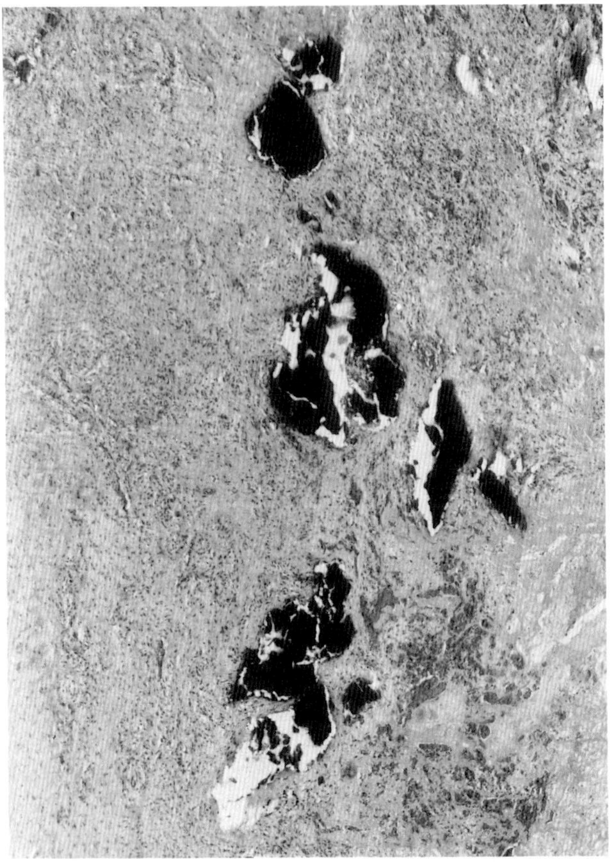

Fig. 78. This 5-year-old thoroughbred gelding fractured both sesamoid bones of the left front limb. The picture shows the left front deep flexor tendon. There is no normal tendon tissue. In the replacing scar tissue are large areas of bone formation (black areas). ×45.

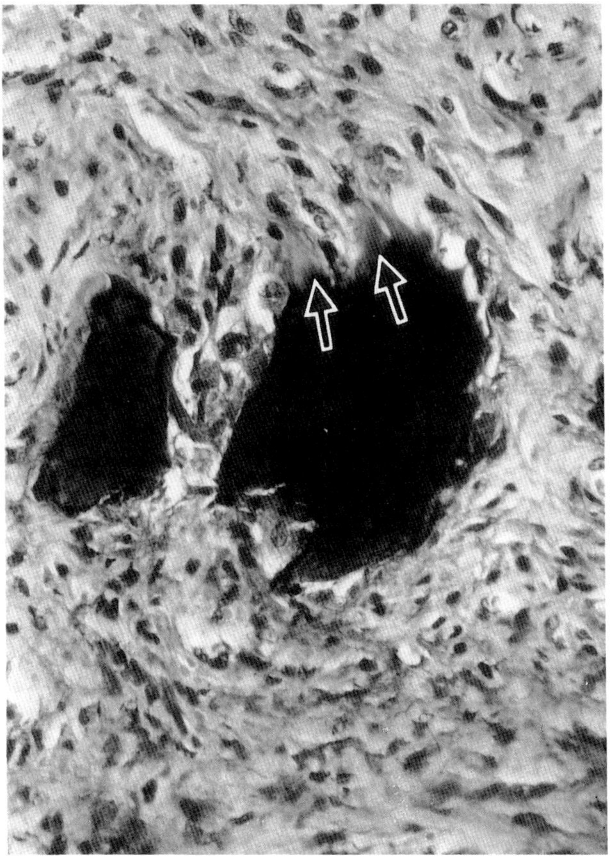

Fig. 79. Same field as in Fig. 78 under higher magnification. The black areas are bone tissue. In front of the arrows are scar tissue cells that have changed to bone-forming cells. ×350.

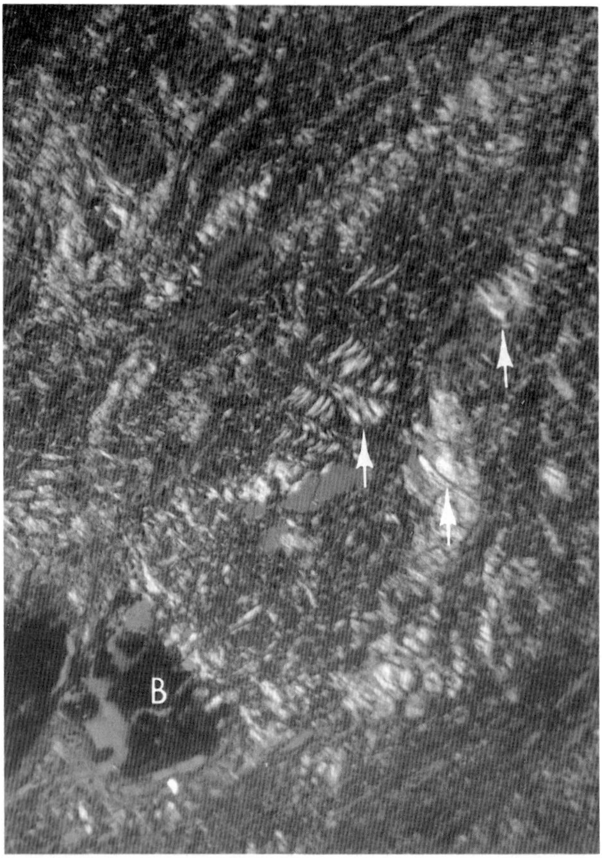

Fig. 80. Same section as in Fig. 78 exposed with polarized light. There are two very small areas of tendon tissue left in front of the arrows. B at the lower left corner is bone (the same bone tissue as in Fig. 79). The rest of the field is occupied by scar tissue. ×120.

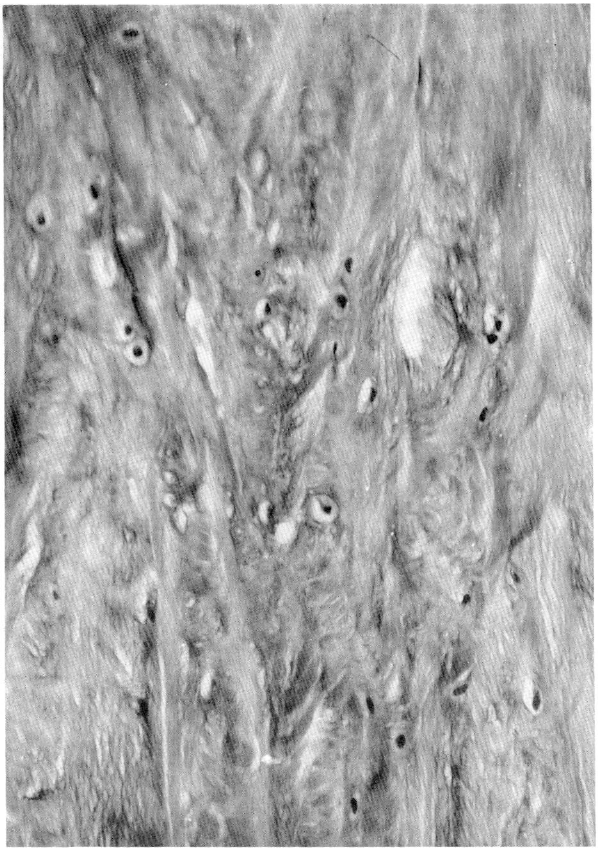

Fig. 81. This 5-year-old thoroughbred stallion fractured the coffin bone of the right hind limb. The picture shows the deep flexor tendon of the right hind limb. There is severe degeneration of the fibers, which are swollen and black by deposition of calcium salts (especially at the lower part). The large, ballooned cells are cartilage cells. ×200.

Fig. 82 and 83. are microscopic pictures of the deep flexor tendon, front limb, of a 2-year-old thoroughbred colt which was fed 400 times the normal amount of vitamin D.

Fig. 82. In a is a lengthwise section of the tendon. The dark areas represent deposits of calcium salts in the tendon. ×45.

In b is a high power microscopic field of a. The dark spots represent calcium deposits in the collagen fibers. ×560.

In c at the left top is an area with calcium salt deposits. Coming in from the lower right are blood vessels with scar tissue. ×110.

In d, at a higher power, the scar tissue cells are removing the calcified tissue (at top) and replacing it with scar tissue. ×450.

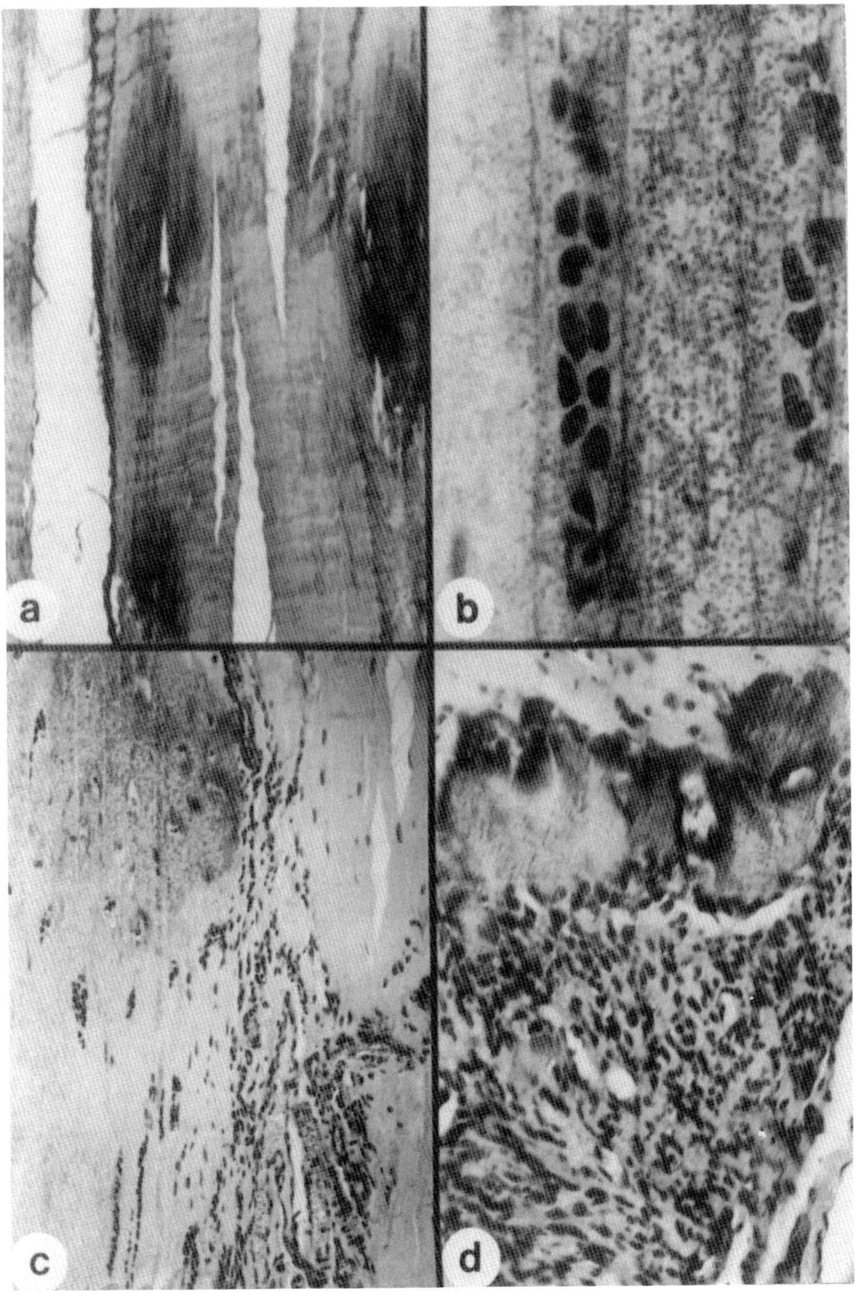
a
b
c
d

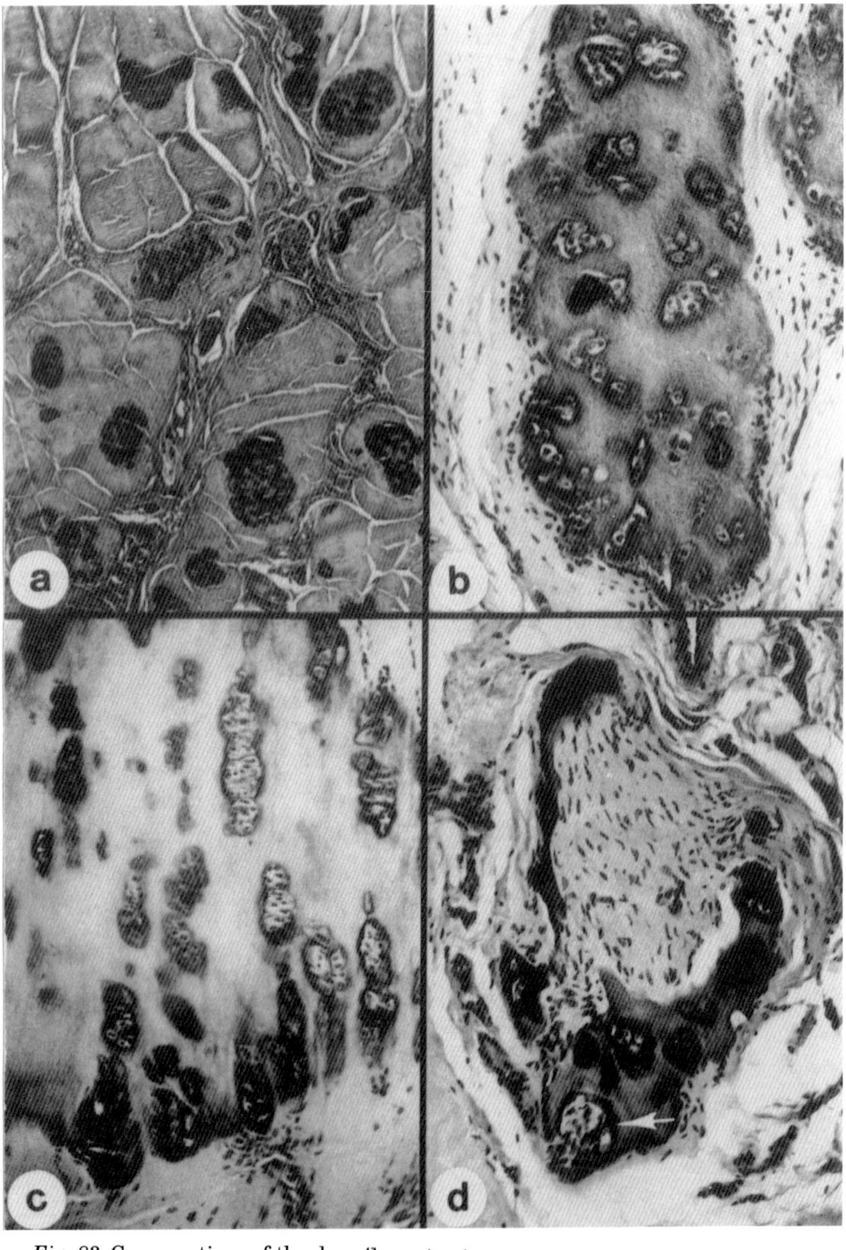

Fig. 83 Cross-sections of the deep flexor tendon.

a. The dark areas represent cartilage formation within the tendon. ×25.

b. One of the dark areas in a is photographed under higher power. ×180. There is formation of cartilage within the tendon.

c. The cartilage cells line up to mimic a growth plate. ×250.

d. Bone is formed beneath the 'growth plate' in c. The bone is being resorbed in front of the arrow at center bottom. ×110.

2. Fractures during races

The distribution of the 53 fractures is shown in Table 9. Fifty cases concerned the front limbs with no left or right preference. The sesamoid bones and the cannon bone accounted for almost two-thirds of all cases. There were 2 cases in the right hind limb and 1 case in a loin back bone.

Table 9. Distribution of fractures

	Left	+ right	= total
Front limb			
Shoulder blade	1	2	3
Arm bone	2	2	4
Forearm + elbow bones	0	0	0
Knee bones	2	6	8
Cannon bone	9	4	13
Sesamoid bones	12	7	19
Long pastern bone	1	1	2
Coffin bone	0	1	1
	27	23	50
Hind limb			
Tibia	0	1	1
Coffin bone	0	1	1
Loin back bone			1
Total	27	25	53

A. *The shoulder blade*

There were 3 cases, all thoroughbred geldings, 2 4-year-olds and 1 7-year-old.

All three fractures started in the lowest part of the shoulder blade and involved the joint cartilage. In two of these cases, gross examination revealed severe OCH changes. Fig. 84 shows one of these cases. The fracture line was directly associated with OCH. The severity of the OCH changes was underscored by a large detached cartilage flap, an OCD.

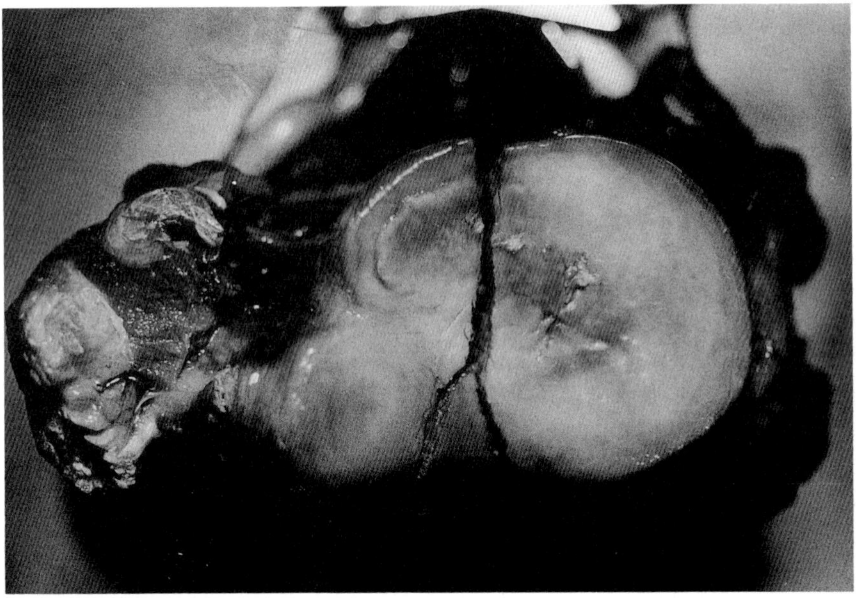

Fig. 84. Thoroughbred gelding, 7-year-old, lower end of right shoulder blade. The front end is to the right; the inner contour is at bottom. There is severe osteochondrosis with a large detached cartilage flap at the inner front end. The fracture line is closely associated with OCH.

In all three cases, the fracture went upward to shatter the neck and body of the shoulder blade. This is called a comminuted fracture, or a fracture in which the bone is crushed into small pieces. The radiographic picture of such a comminuted fracture of the shoulder blade appears in Fig. 85.

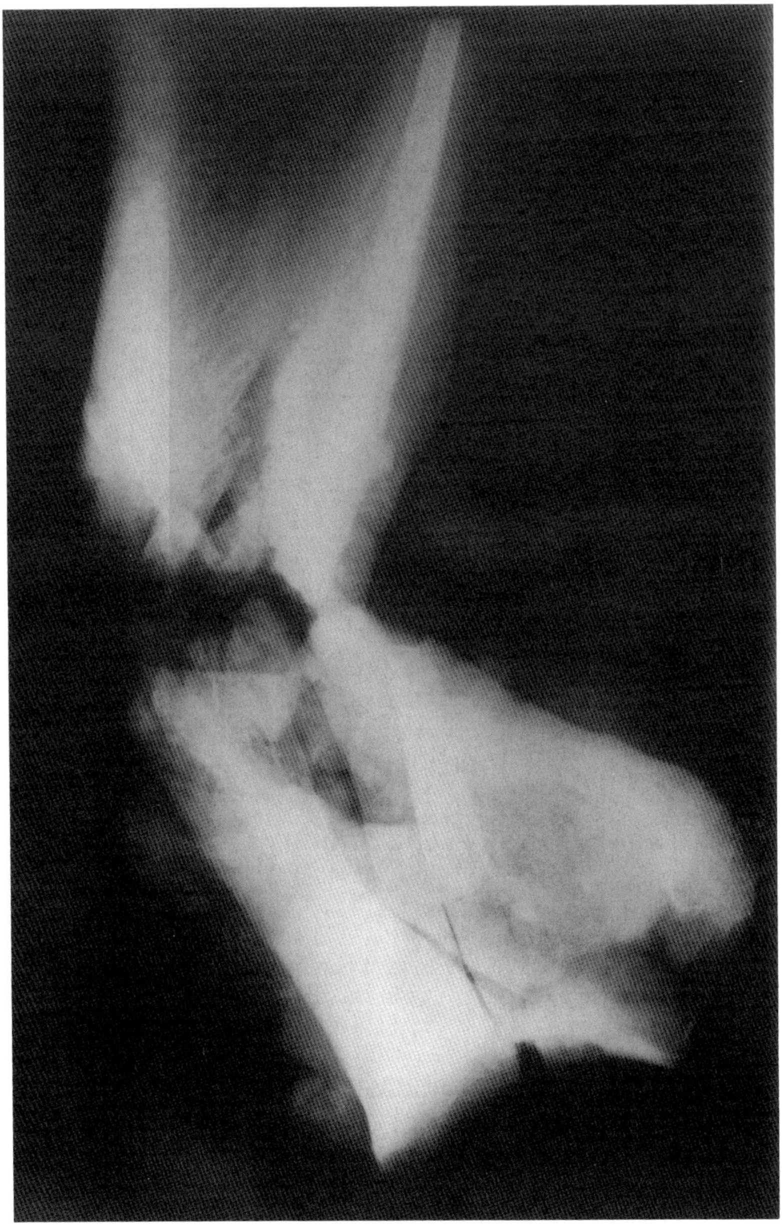

Fig. 85. Same horse as in Fig. 84. Radiograph of the right shoulder blade from outside. The fracture starts at the articular cartilage and goes upward to shatter the bone.

Fig. 86 shows a microscopic view of the lower end of the shoulder blade of the case in Figs. 84 and 85. The OCH changes in the cartilage itself are obvious. More important are the changes in the bone beneath the cartilage. The bone plate beneath the joint cartilage fails to form, a failure that constitutes the weak point through which the fracture occurs.

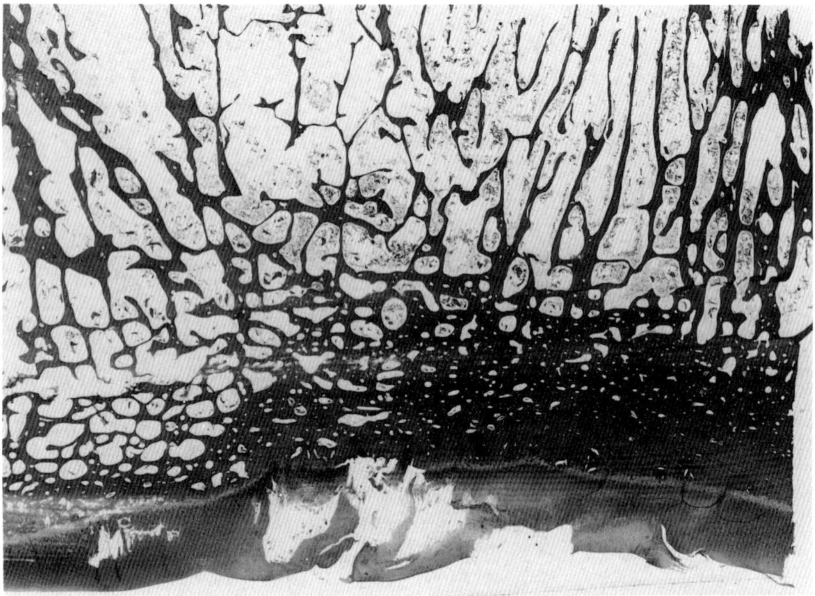

Fig. 86. Same horse as in Fig. 84. This microscopic section is taken parallel to the fracture line. To the right is a thick bone plate beneath the joint cartilage. Going to the left, the plate becomes thinner and disappears. The bone bars beneath the joint cartilage to the left are arranged horizontally. The cartilage presents huge defects. ×3.5.

In another case of shoulder-blade fracture, the gross changes of OCH were almost identical to those of the first case just described. The lack of formation of a bone plate beneath the joint cartilage is illustrated in Fig. 87.

In the third case, there were no gross changes in the joint cartilage of the shoulder blade. Radiographs of slab sections parallel to the fracture line showed changes closely similar to those shown in Fig. 87.

In conclusion, the three fractures of the shoulder blade resulted from OCH. Thus, the fractures are pathological.

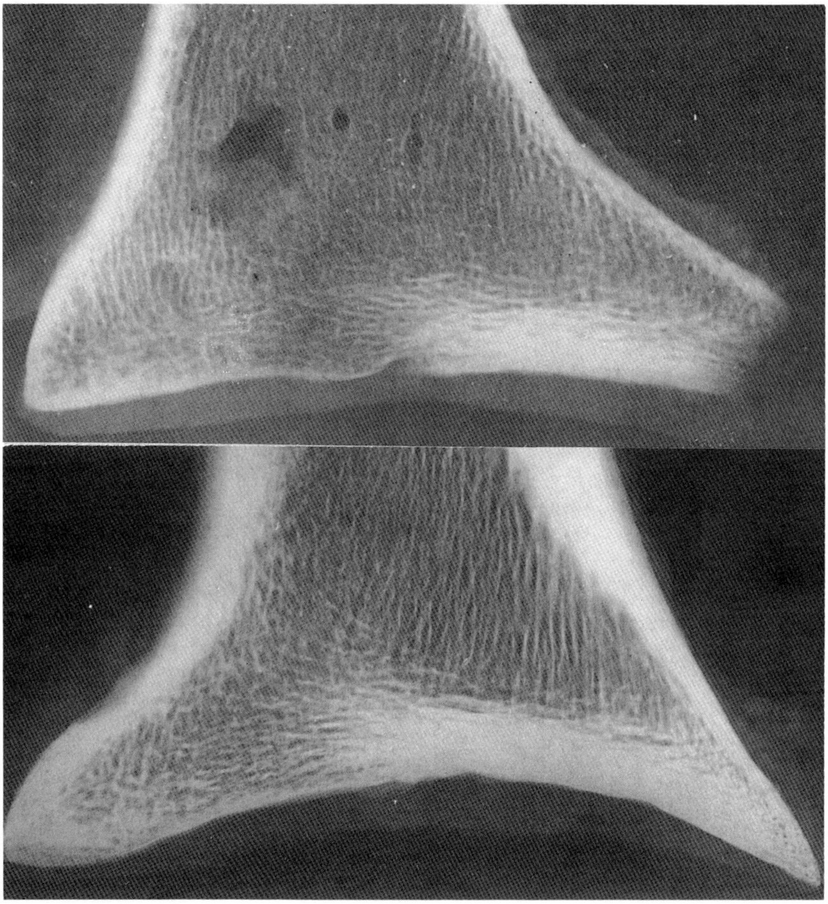

Fig. 87. A 4-year-old thoroughbred gelding, radiographs of slab sections parallel to the fracture. The bone plate is well defined to the right but disappears toward the left. Note that the bone bars at the areas of missing bone plate are arranged horizontally. ×2.

B. *The arm bone*

There were 4 cases, 3 stallions and 1 gelding. Three horses were 5-year-old and 1 was 6-year-old.

Two cases concerned the upper end, one the lower end; one was a spiral fracture of the shaft.

In the first case of fracture of the upper end, the fracture line detached the inner third of the head of the arm bone (the lesser tubercle). As shown in Fig. 88, the fracture line was closely associated with severe OCH. A radiograph of a slab section parallel to the fracture line revealed two large cysts beneath the joint cartilage (Fig. 89).

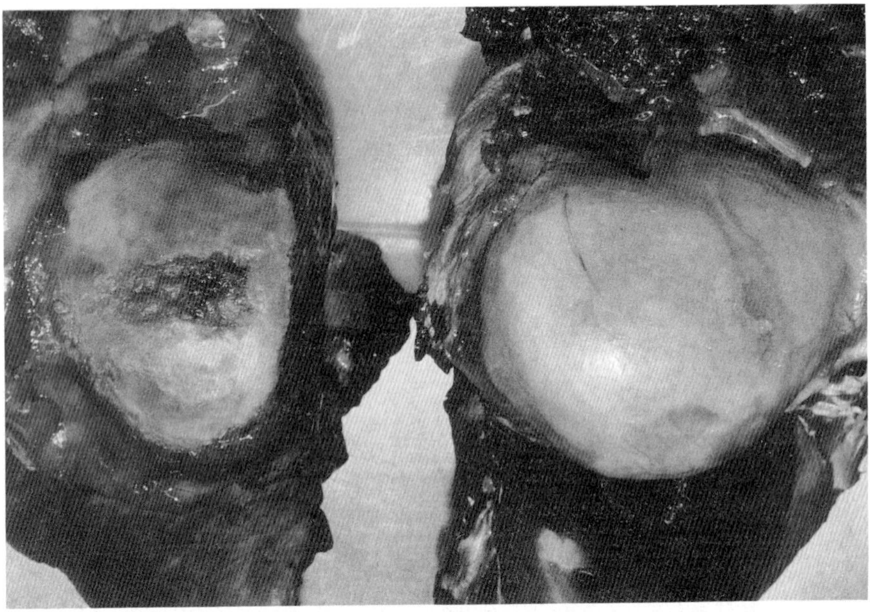

Fig. 88. A 6-year-old thoroughbred stallion. Heads of the arm bones are seen from behind. The fracture has detached the inner third (the lesser tubercle) of the head of the left arm bone. There is severe OCH of the head of that bone.

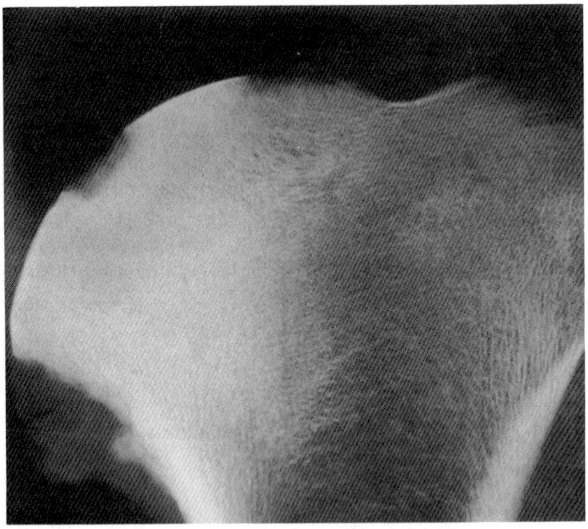

Fig. 89. Radiograph of slab section parallel to the fracture shown in Fig. 88. The back contour of the head of the arm bone is to the left. There are two deep cysts beneath the joint cartilage. Note also that the bone in the left part is much denser than normal.

It should be noted that this radiograph also showed very dense bone (osteopetrosis) in the back half of the head of the arm bone.

The second case closely resembled the first, except that the right arm bone had fractured (Fig. 90). Again, the fracture occurred because of OCH (Figs. 91 and 92). On gross examination (Fig. 91), there was severe OCH even with OCD, and radiography of a slab section showed

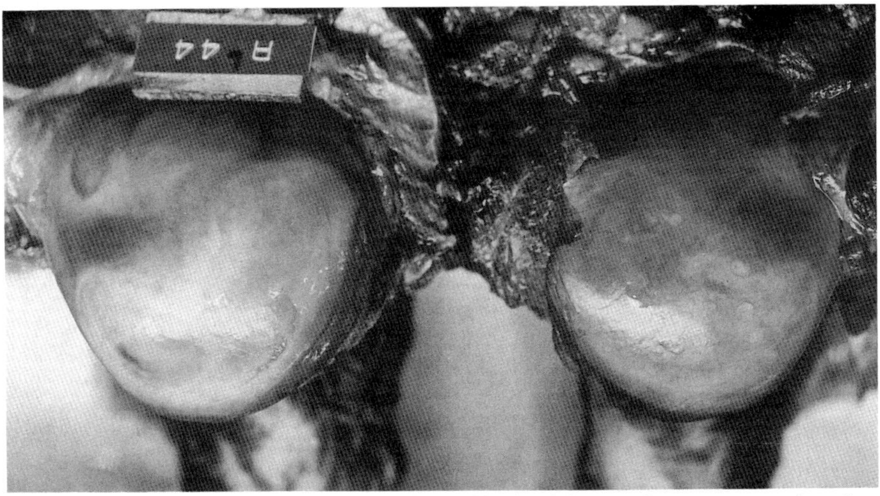

Fig. 90. A 5-year-old thoroughbred stallion. Heads of the arm bones are seen from behind. The fracture has detached the inner fourth (the lesser tubercle) of the head of the right arm bone. There is extensive OCH of the head of that bone.

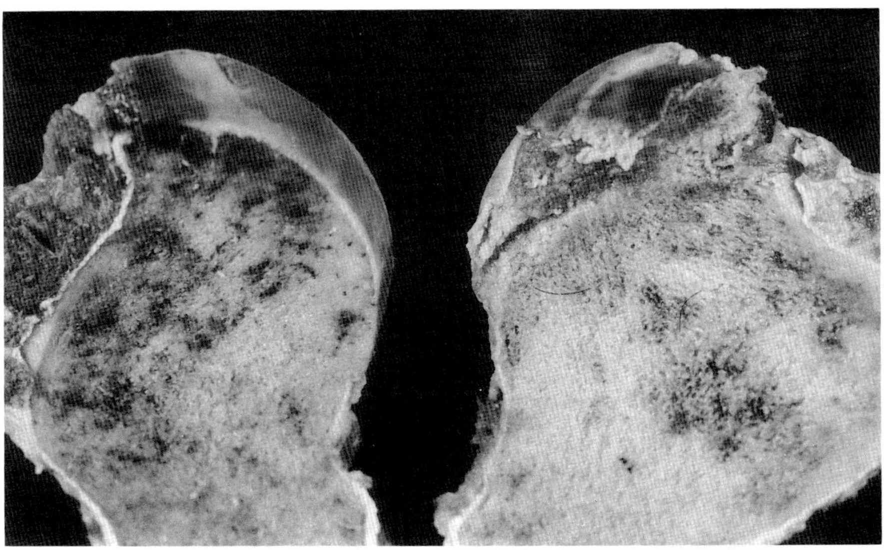

Fig. 91. Section cut parallel to the fracture of the head of the right arm bone and at a similar site on the head of the left arm bone. Note the severe OCH and OCD of the right head.

that the fracture occurred through multiple cysts (Figs. 92). The microscopic picture (Figs. 93 and 94) showed classic examples of OCH. The joint cartilage was severely frayed, and there were cracks between the joint cartilage and the underlying bone (Fig. 93). Large areas of retained cartilage occurred beneath the joint cartilage, areas

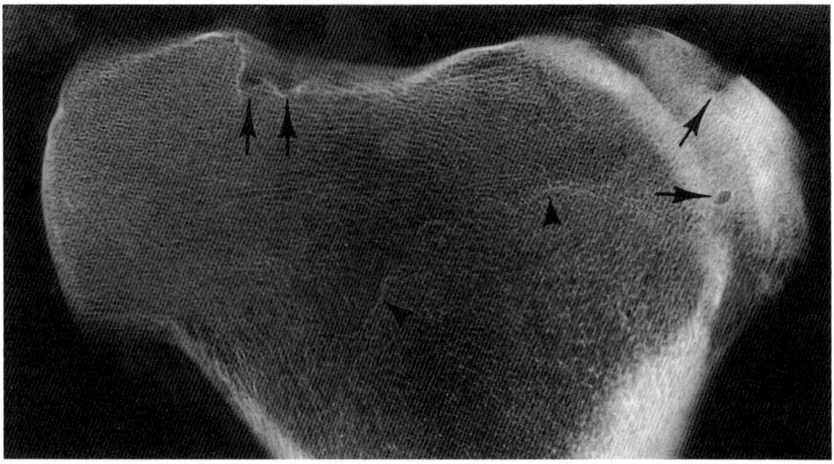

Fig. 92. Radiograph of slab section parallel to the fracture shown in Fig. 90. In front of the arrows are cysts beneath the joint cartilage. The white line in front of arrowhead is the last remnant of the growth plate.

that formed neither the subchondral plate nor the bone bars (trabeculae) in the head of this arm bone. Under higher miscroscopic enlargement (Fig. 94), the failure of cartilage to convert into bone, our definition of OCH, caused total chaos of cartilage and bone with none of the tissues arranged to perform normal functions. Cracks occurred within such retained cartilage and between cartilage and bone tissues. Such chaotic arrangement of cartilage and bone, the presence of subchondral cysts, and frayed and cracked joint cartilage are perfect reasons for a fracture to occur.

The third case concerned the lower end of the arm bone. The radiograph of the post-mortem specimen (Fig. 95) showed a classical example of a comminuted fracture. The microscopic examination tells why this happened. We see in Fig. 96 the lower end of one of the shattered large pieces. The joint cartilage is very thin and pale. There is no bone plate beneath the joint cartilage, which in many areas faces soft tissue rather than bone. The bone bars are thin and arranged transversely. Compared to Figs. 23 and 24 in Chapter III, the joint area in Fig. 96 is one of very little strength; this weak area is the cause of the horse's fracture.

The fourth case was a spiral fracture of the shaft with no involvement of either end. Thus, OCH cannot be expected and was not found.

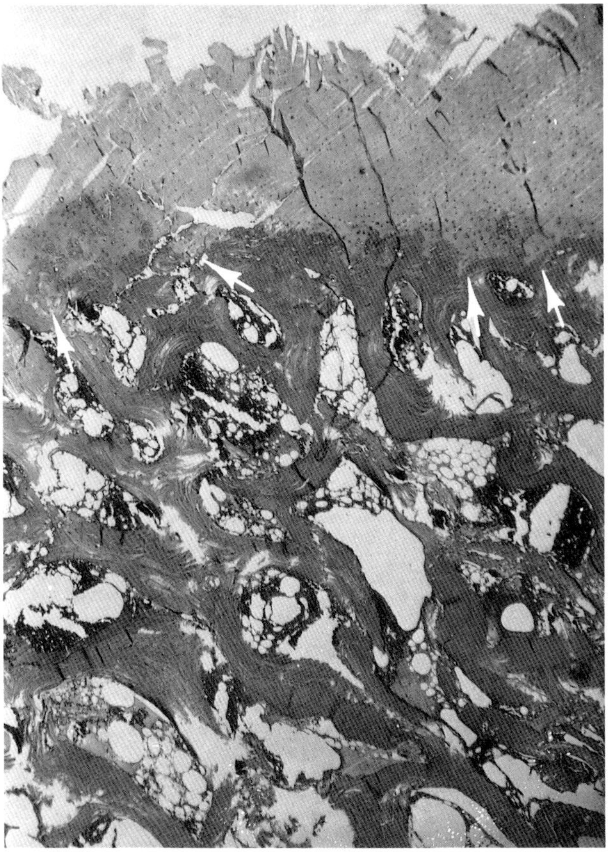

Fig. 93. A microscopic section of the head of the arm bone next to the fracture shown in Fig. 90. The joint cartilage at top is severely frayed and cracked. In front of arrows are areas of retained cartilage that do not form a subchondral bone plate or bone bars. ×25.

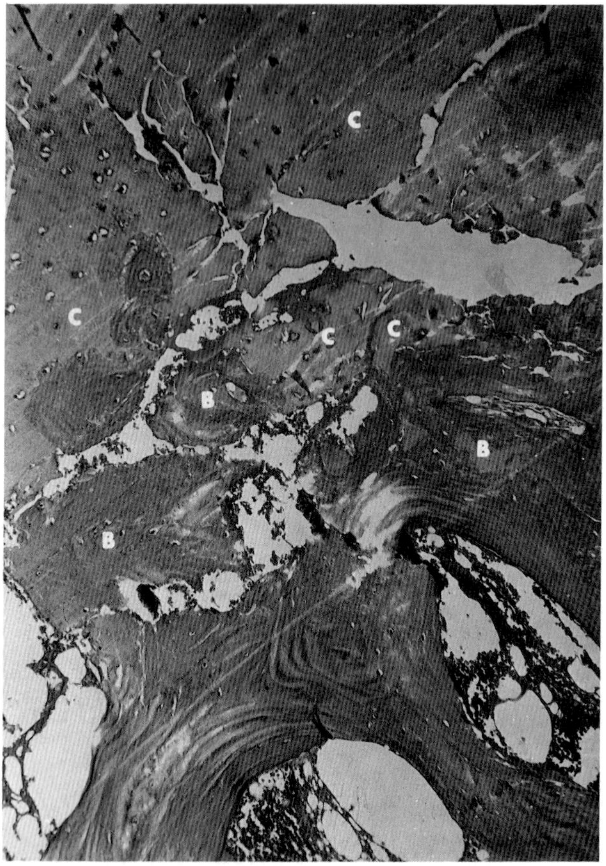

Fig. 94. This is a higher magnification of the field in front of the second arrow from the left in Fig. 93. Retained cartilage (c) is chaotically mixed up with bone tissue (b). There are cracks within cartilage and between cartilage and bone. ×100.

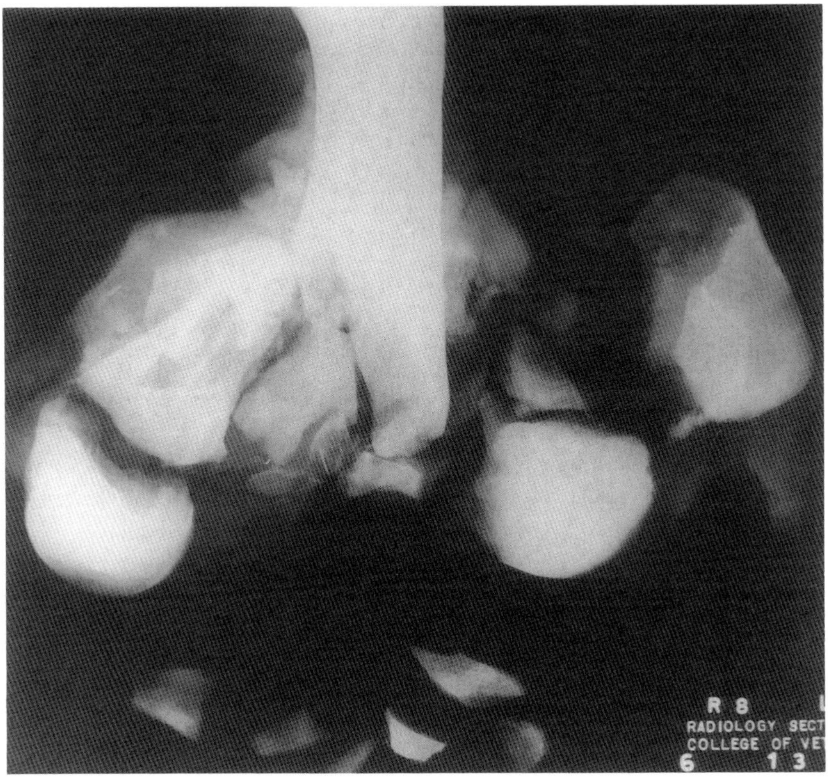

Fig. 95. This figure shows a radiograph of the lower end of the left arm bone of a 5-year-old thoroughbred stallion. The lower end is shattered into numerous large and small pieces.

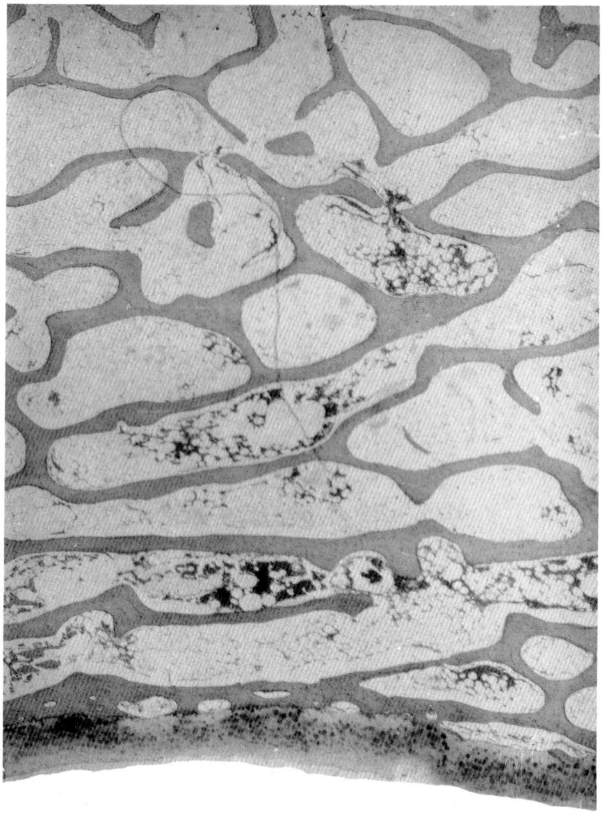

Fig. 96. This is a microscopic section through one of the larger pieces from the fracture shown in Fig. 95. At bottom is the joint cartilage, which is very thin, pale, and devoid of bone beneath. The bone bars are thin and arranged transversely. ×18.

No other changes were recorded to explain the fracture. If bone or cartilage changes *are* found, we are dealing with a pathological fracture. If such changes are not found, a pathologic fracture cannot be excluded, because the absense of such changes may simply mean that the appropriate tissues to demonstrate the changes were not collected and examined. A positive finding is diagnostic, but a negative finding is not exclusive.

C. *The knee bones*

There were 8 cases: 3 colts, 2 fillies and 2 geldings. One filly fractured both knees, producing two cases from one filly. All were 3-year-olds, except the one 4-year-old. There were 10 bones fractured in the upper row and 15 in the lower row.

All fractures were pathologic, and the underlying diseases were OCH and CON. In one case, OCH was the immediate cause of the fracture. OCH occurred in the other cases, but not to a degree to explain the fracture. In these 7 cases, CON was considered to be the most important change.

The severe OCH case was a 4-year-old thoroughbred gelding that fractured the inner bone of the upper row on the right side (radial knee bone) and the inner and central bone of the lower row (2nd and 3rd knee bones, respectively). The gross and radiographic pictures of the fractures in the lower row bones are shown in Figs. 97 and 98,

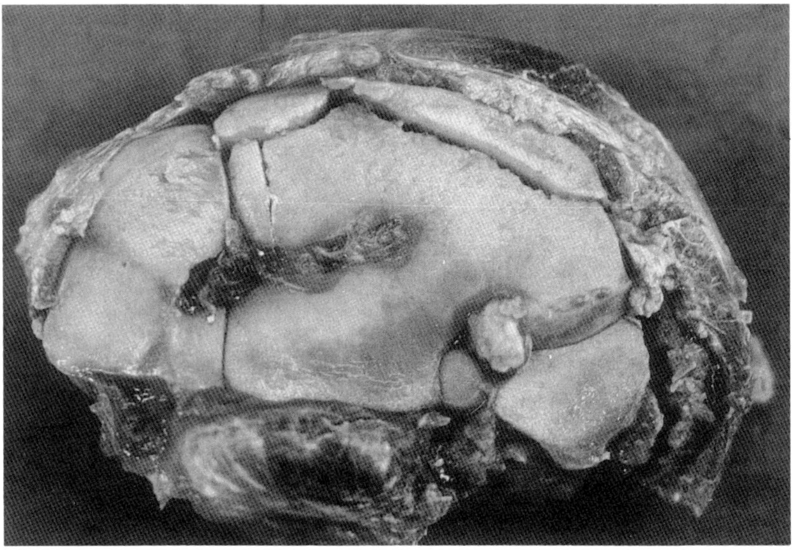

Fig. 97. A 4-year-old thoroughbred gelding. The picture shows the lower row of knee bones seen from below. The large middle bone (the 3rd knee bone) is fractured into 3 pieces. The outer right knee bone (4th knee bone to the lower right) is also fractured. There is a deep transverse ditch in the joint cartilage of the 3rd knee bone.

respectively. Though the pictures tell where the fractures are, they do not tell why they are there. The gross picture (Fig. 97) shows an OCH change in the 3rd knee bone but that change is not directly associated with the fracture. So again, we must examine the bones under the microscope. In Fig. 99 is a section of the 3rd knee bone. The section includes the main part of the 3rd knee bone and starts just inside the fracture line and extends backward. The fracture goes through a large area of scar tissue which replaces the previous cyst. Several more cysts filled with retained and degenerate cartilage are present in the field. Further back in the same section is a large piece of retained cartilage that has not yet degenerated to form a cyst (Fig. 100). The retained cartilage is pale and contains very few cells. The border to

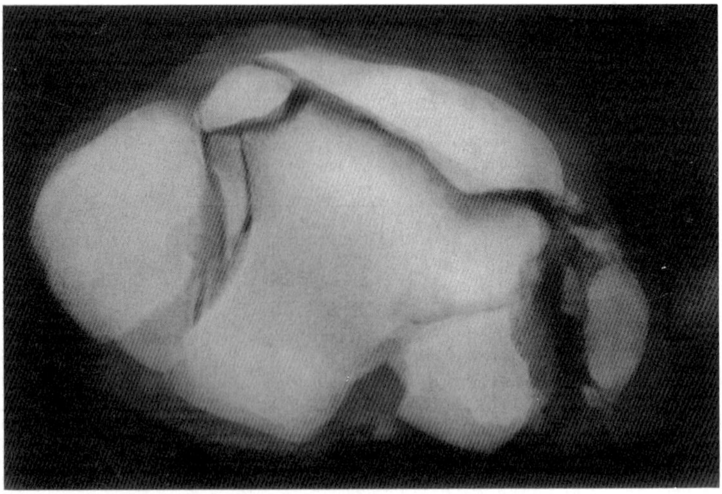

Fig. 98. This is a radiograph of the specimen presented in Fig. 97. The fracture lines are more easily noted in the radiograph.

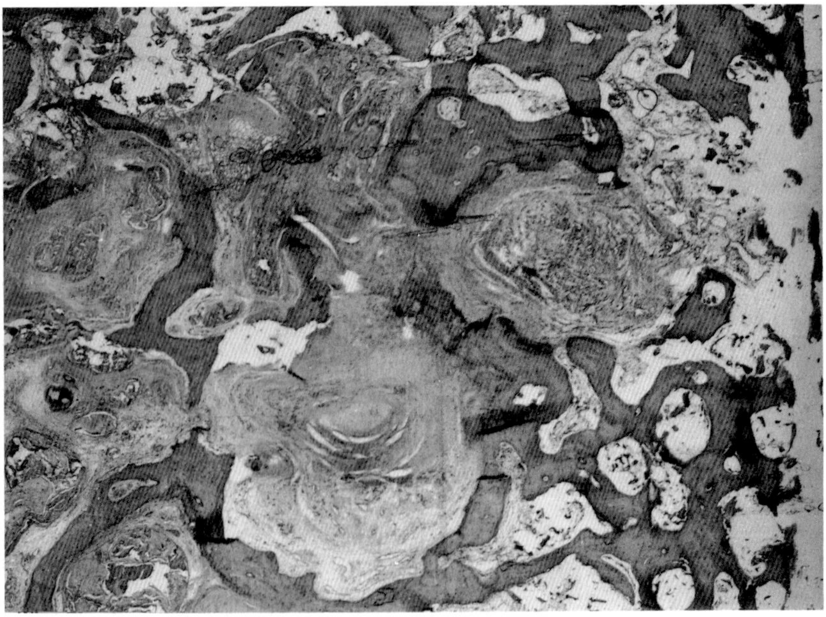

Fig. 99. This is a microscopic section from front to back through the fractured 3rd knee bone in Fig. 98. The fracture line is to the far right and goes through a cyst. There are 4 additional cysts formed in retained cartilage. ×18.

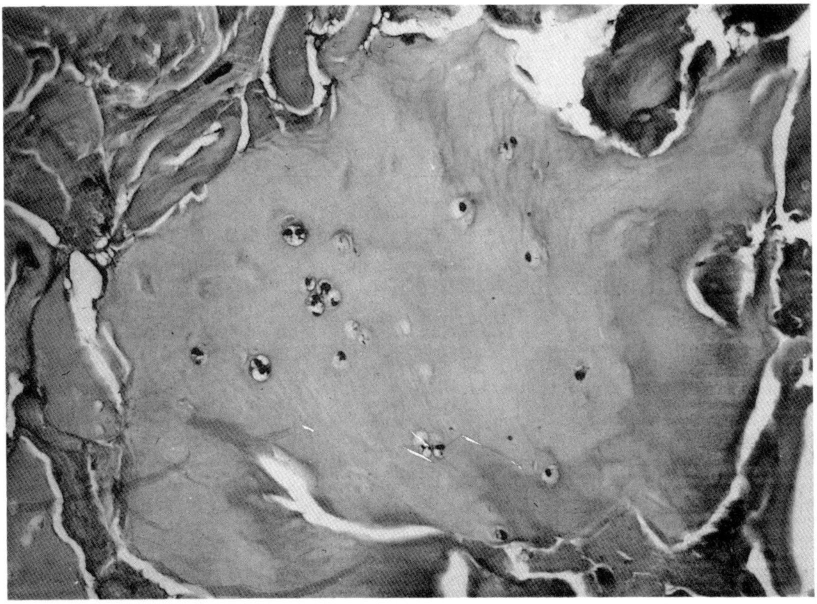

Fig. 100. Same microscopic section as in Fig. 98, taken a little further back. There is a huge chunk of cartilage retained within the 3rd knee bone. The cartilage has few cells and is pale. The border to surrounding bone is sharp, and there is no other tissue between cartilage and bone. ×180.

surrounding bone tissue is sharp with no intervening tissue. All changes shown in Figs. 99 and 100 are clear-cut examples of OCH, a failure of cartilage to convert to bone.

Cartilage within bone can occur for another reason, namely in healing of a fracture. In a healing fracture, scar tissue is formed between the adjacent bone tissues. Cartilage is formed within the scar tissue, and the cartilage is eventually converted into bone. The events in fracture healing differ markedly from those in retained cartilage. As shown in Fig. 101, fracture healing cartilage is stained darkly and contains a large amount of densely packed cells. Furthermore, there is usually a rim of scar tissue between cartilage and bone.

Now to the CON changes. Figs. 102-107 are from a 3-year-old thoroughbred gelding that fractured two bones of the upper and lower rows of right knee bones. Fig. 102 presents the upper row seen from above. The fracture of the inner (radial knee bone, to the left) and of the outer (ulnar knee bone) knee bones are easily recognized, but the joint cartilages present no remarkable changes. Seen from below (Fig. 102), the bones show most convincing changes. There is very extensive destruction of the joint cartilage of the inner and middle knee bones with exposure of the underlying bone. The fracture of the inner bone goes straight through the extensive change of CON. The fractures of

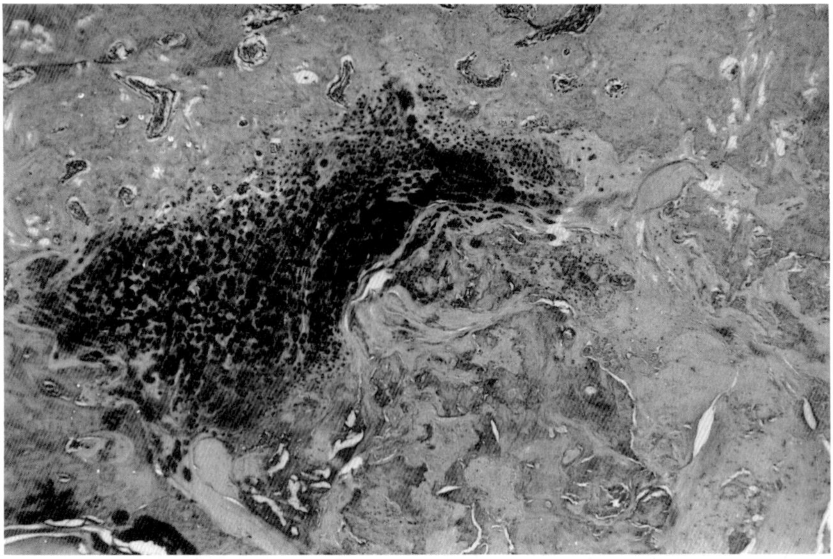

Fig. 101. This is a microscopic section through the left 3rd knee bone of the horse described in Fig. 66. The large dark area represents cartilage formed as part of the healing of a fracture. There are numerous cells within this cartilage, and there is a soft-tissue junction between this cartilage and the surrounding bone. ×30.

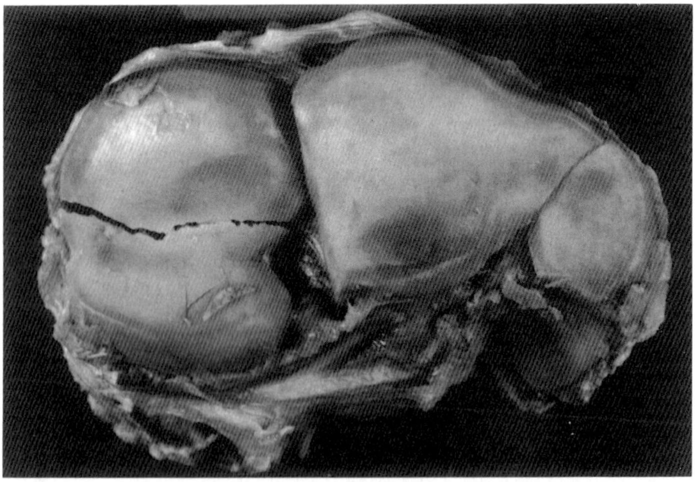

Fig. 102. A 3-year-old thoroughbred gelding that fractured two bones of the upper row knee bones and three of the lower row of the right knee. The picture shows the upper row seen from above. There is a transverse fracture of the inner knee bone (radial knee bone). The joint cartilages show no remarkable changes.

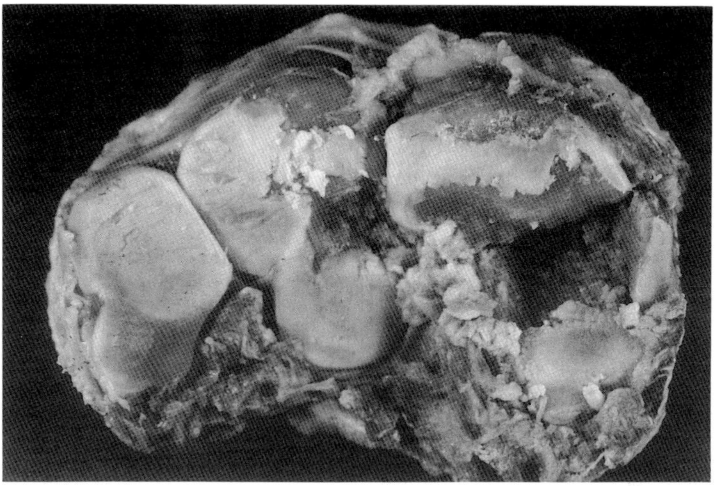

Fig. 103. Same horse as in Fig. 102. The upper row of knee bones is seen from below. There is very severe chondro-osteo-necrosis (CON) of the inner row (radial knee bone) and of the middle (intermediate knee bone) with exposure of the underlying bone. The transverse fracture of the inner knee bone goes through this CON. Compare with Fig. 102.

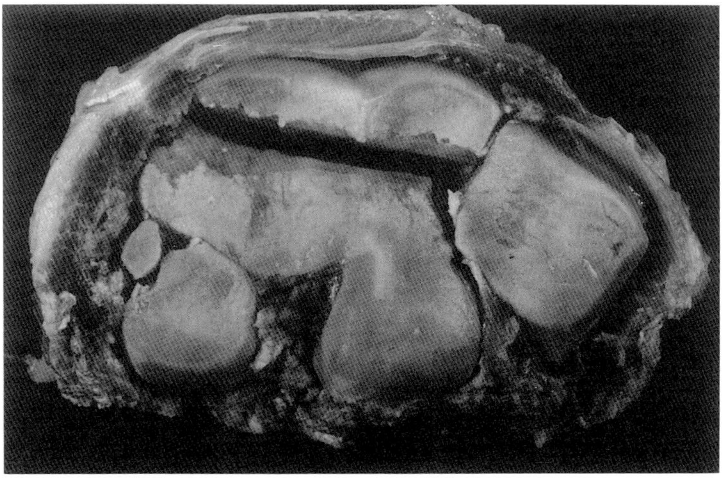

Fig. 104. Same horse as in Fig. 102. The lower row of knee bones is seen from above. There is a fracture of the front part of the 3rd knee bone (middle) and of the front inner part of the 2nd knee bone (middle left). There is cartilage destruction around the fracture of the 3rd bone.

the lower bone row are shown in Fig. 104 (from above) and in Fig. 105 (from below). There is cartilage destruction associated with the fracture of the knee bone (Fig. 104) but whether this is due to shattering during the fracture or to changes in the cartilage cannot be stated from gross inspection. Minor changes of CON were observed in the

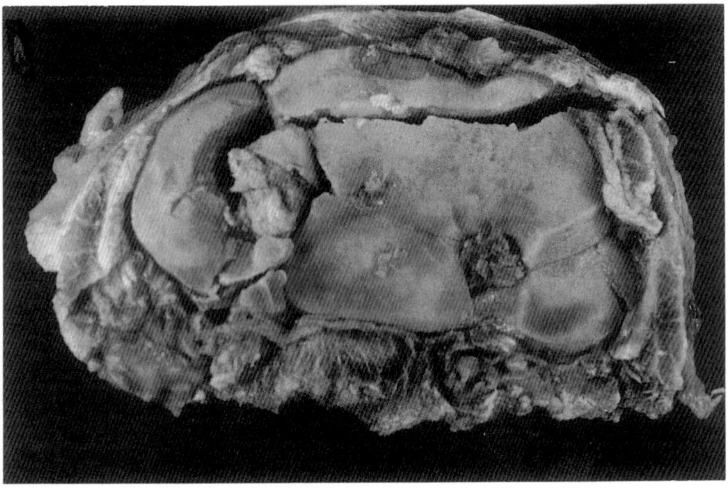

Fig. 105. Same horse as in Fig. 102. The lower row of knee bones are seen from below. The fractures seen from above in Fig. 106 go vertically through the bones.

microscope which could have contributed to the fractures. The fractures of the lower row bones could, possibly, occur as a result of the fracture of the upper row bones.

The middle bone of the upper right row (intermediate knee bone), the gross changes of which appear in Fig. 103, will now be shown under the microscope. The figures (106 and 107) show the cartilage is pale and contains few cells. These changes become worse in the middle and upper part of the picture. These changes signify death of the cartilage which is falling apart. The tight junction to the underlying bone is lost, and the bone also dies. The changes are still better demonstrated in Fig. 107. The surface cartilage is frayed, cartilage cells are disappearing, and at the cartilage-to-bone junction, both tissues are dead.

The CON changes are not restricted to the knee bones that fractured. Adjoining bones are also affected. Fig. 108 shows the lower end of the right forearm bone of a 3-year-old thoroughbred filly that fractured both knees. In the left knee, there were 5 fractures, 2 of the upper row and 3 of the lower row, and in the right knee there were 4 fractures, 2 bones in each row. The knee bones showed, under the microscope, definite CON changes of the lower end of both forearms. Fig. 108 shows very severe CON changes in the lower part of the right forearm.

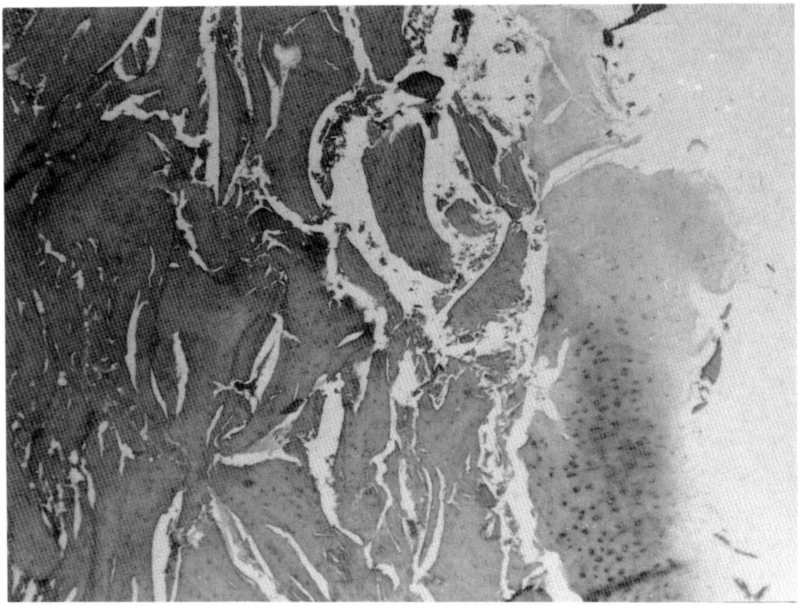

Fig. 106. Same horse as in Fig. 102. To the right is the joint cartilage of the middle bone of the upper row of the right knee (intermediate knee bone). The lower part is pale and the cells are relatively few. These changes grow worse, and in the middle the cartilage is very pale with only a few cells. At top, the cartilage is dead and is falling apart. Beneath the cartilage is severe necrosis of the bone. ×40.

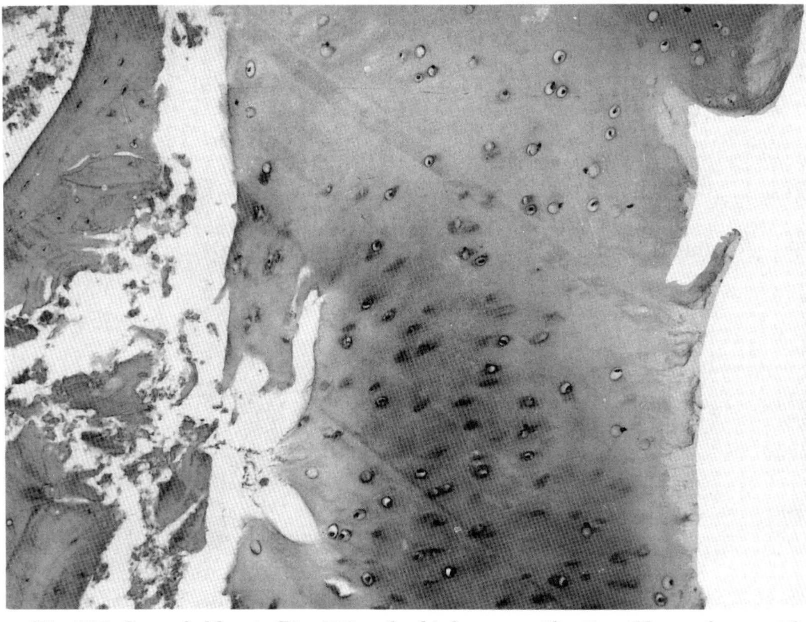

Fig. 107. Same field as in Fig. 106 under higher magnification. The surface cartilage is frayed, the cartilage is pale with few cells and is falling apart in its inner part. The underlying bone is dead. ×120.

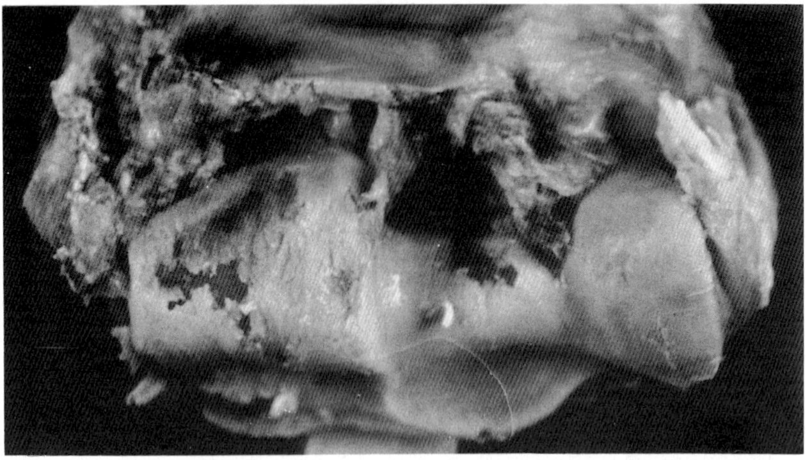

Fig. 108. A 3-year-old thoroughbred filly which fractured both knees, 5 bones in the left knee, and 4 in the right. The picture shows the lower end of the right forearm bone seen slightly from behind. There is severe, extensive CON.

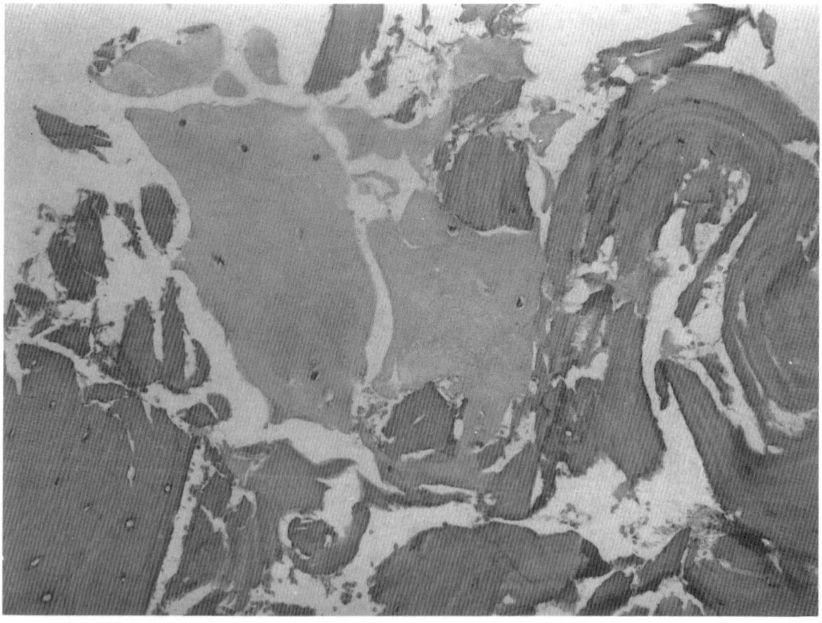

Fig. 109. Same filly as in Fig. 108. This is a microscopic picture through the right inner bone (radial knee bone) of the upper row. In the center are two large chunks of fetal bone that did not convert into bone. The surrounding bone is shattered. ×180.

As stated above, the knee bones showed a mixture of OCH and CON changes. In the case in Fig. 108, the inner right bone of the upper row presented the microscopic changes shown in Fig. 109. There are two lumps of retained fetal cartilage that have no functional correlation to the surrounding, shattered bone.

We will return to the interaction of OCH and CON in the next chapter.

Whatever the reason for knee bone fracture, OCH or CON, the fractures studied are pathological.

D. *The cannon bone*

There were 13 cases: 6 colts, 2 fillies, 4 geldings, and 1 stallion. The ages were 7 3-year-olds, 3 4-year-olds, 2 5-year-olds, and 1 10-year-old. The fractures started in the upper end in 4 cases, in the lower end in 4 cases, and in 1 case both ends were involved. In all but 1 of these cases, the shaft was involved. Only the shaft was involved in 5 cases.

We begin the description with a 3-year-old thoroughbred colt that fractured the upper end and the shaft of the left cannon bone (Figs. 110 and 111). The upper end presented a comminuted fracture (Fig. 110). The joint cartilage showed no remarkable changes other than the fractures. The microscopic picture of a section parallel to one of the

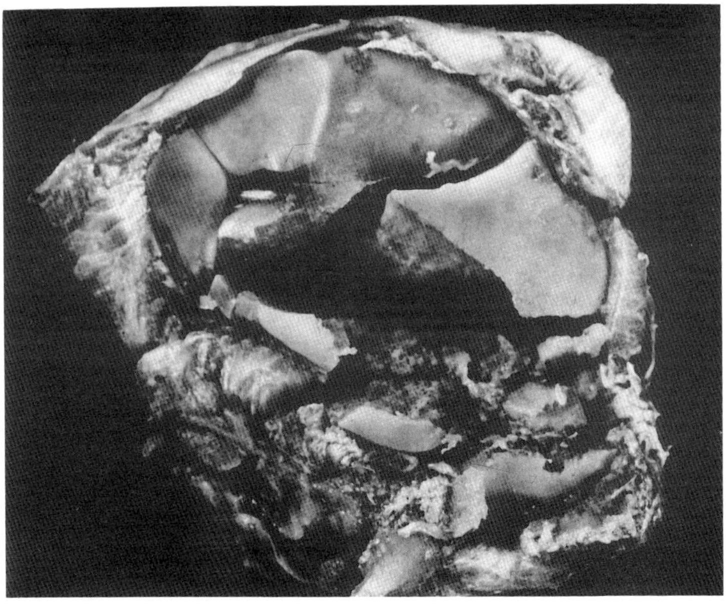

Fig. 110. A 3-year-old thoroughbred colt. This figure shows the upper end of the left front cannon bone. There is a comminuted fracture. Note that there are no signs of OCH.

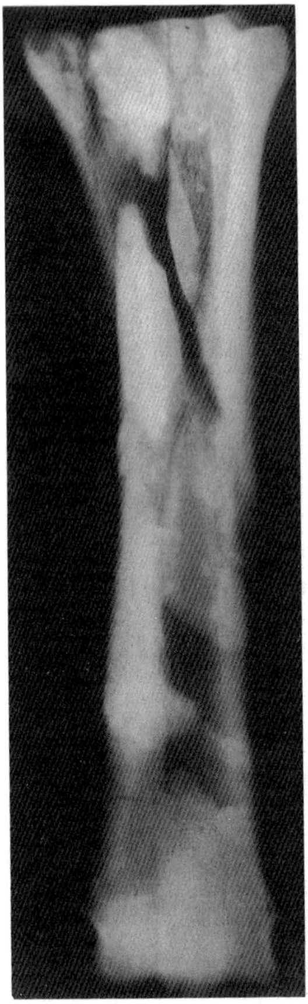

Fig. 111. Same horse as in Fig. 110, this time in a radiograph of the left front cannon bone. There is a comminuted fracture involving the upper end and the shaft but not the lower end.

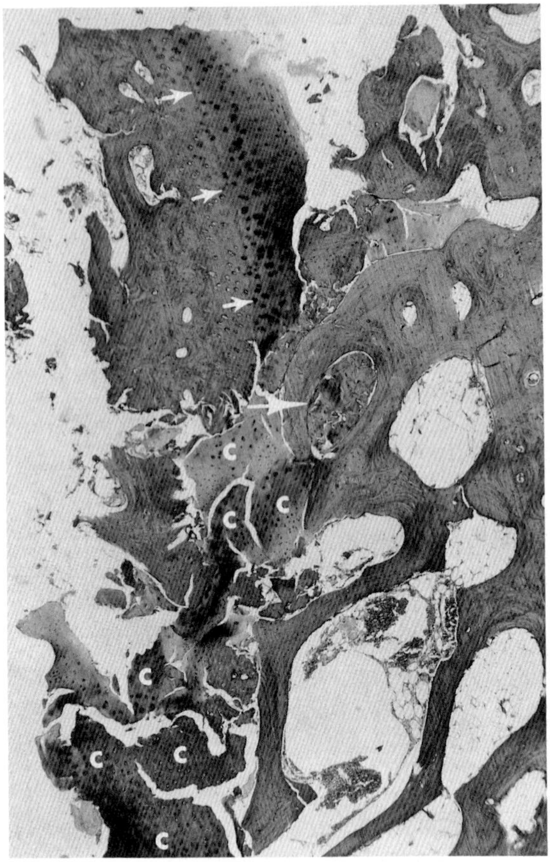

Fig. 112. Same horse as in Fig. 110, microscopic section of the upper end of the cannon bone parallel to one fracture line. The structure in front of the white small arrows represents joint cartilage displaced during the fracture. The areas marked c represent retained fetal cartilage. The large white arrow points to an area within the retained cartilage where bone has been formed. ×25.

fracture lines through the upper end (Fig. 112) shows that the joint cartilage was displaced during the fracture and that this piece of cartilage showed normal dark staining and had a normal, thick subchondral plate. Deeper in this section are several pieces of cartilage (Fig. 112) that, under higher microscopic magnification (Fig. 113), clearly are retained fetal cartilage. This cartilage is pale and contains relatively few cells. It has no connection to the surrounding bone. A small area of bone is formed within this retained cartilage.

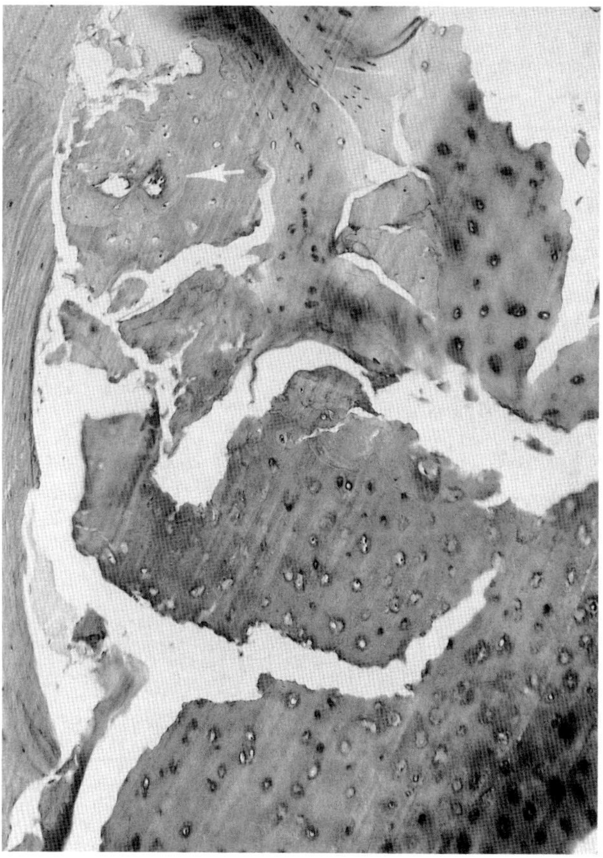

Fig. 113. Same field as in Fig. 112 under higher microscopic magnification. Most of the field is occupied by retained fetal cartilage, which is pale and contains relatively few cells. The cartilage has no connection with bone tissue. In front of the arrow is a small island of bone formed within the fetal cartilage. ×100.

The next case is a 3-year-old thoroughbred gelding that fractured the left cannon bone (Fig. 114). On gross examination, the fracture involves the shaft, is comminuted, and has caused a large wound through the skin. This is called an open or compound fracture. A radiograph of the cannon bone showed that the fracture started at the upper end and split the top in the midline from front to back. There were no remarkable gross changes in the joint cartilage. In Fig. 115 we have a radiograph of a slab section parallel to the fracture line. The subchondral bone plate is well developed at the front and back ends, but in the center it is absent. There is a minimal amount of bone in this area, and the thin trabeculae are arranged transversely. This is also most evident in the microscopic sections (Fig. 116). Note that

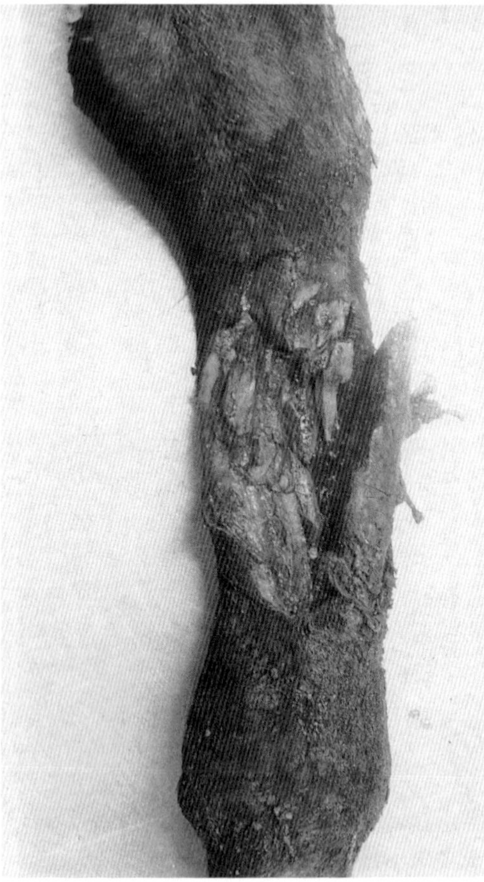

Fig. 114. A 3-year-old thoroughbred gelding that fractured the left cannon bone. The fracture is compound.

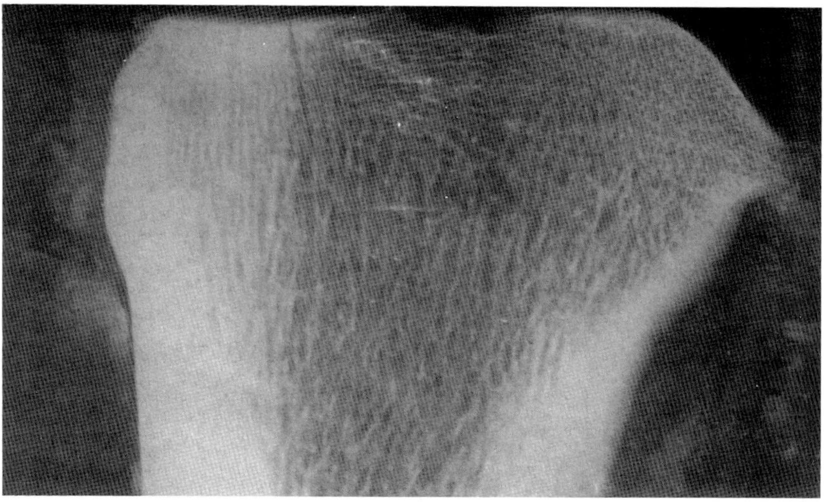

Fig. 115. Same horse as in Fig. 114. This radiograph shows slab section parallel to the fracture of the upper end of the left cannon bone. Front end is to the left. In the top middle third is very little bone, no subchondral bone plate, and pronounced transverse trabeculation. The front and back ends show denser-than-normal bone (osteopetrosis).

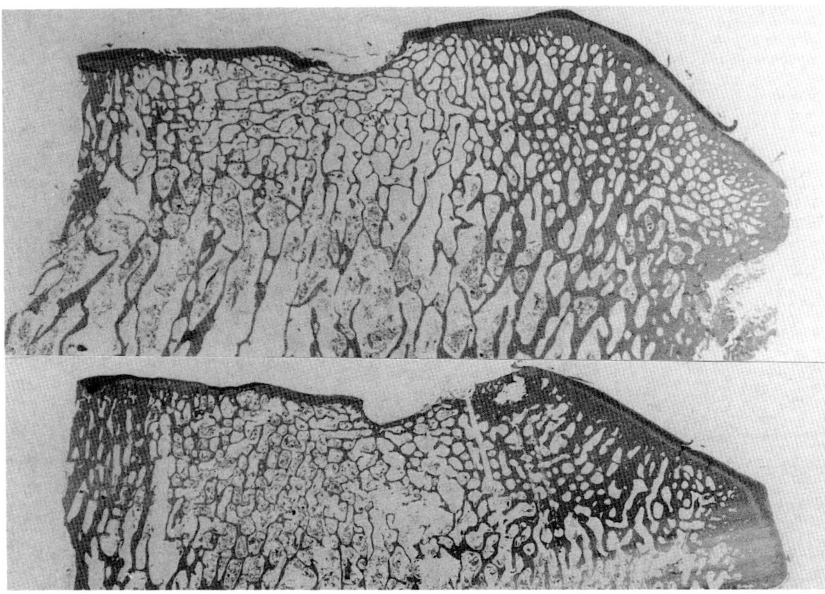

Fig. 116. Same horse as in Fig. 114. Microscopic sections parallel to the fracture through the upper end of the left cannon bone. The front end is to the left. In the top center in both sections is thin cartilage. There is very little bone beneath the cartilage with no defined subchondral plate. The trabeculae are arranged transversely. In the lower section is a cyst beneath the highest point of the cartilage. The back end corners (to the right) show moderate osteopetrosis. ×2.6.

there is a bone cyst beneath the joint cartilage. As seen both in the radiograph of the slab section (Fig. 115) and in the microscopic sections (Fig. 116), the front and back ends present denser than normal bone, or osteopetrosis.

In another case, a 3-year-old thoroughbred filly fractured her right cannon bone. The fracture involved both ends and the shaft (Fig. 117). The fracture was comminuted and compound. In the radiograph (Fig. 117), the pieces were left as they were after the fracture by

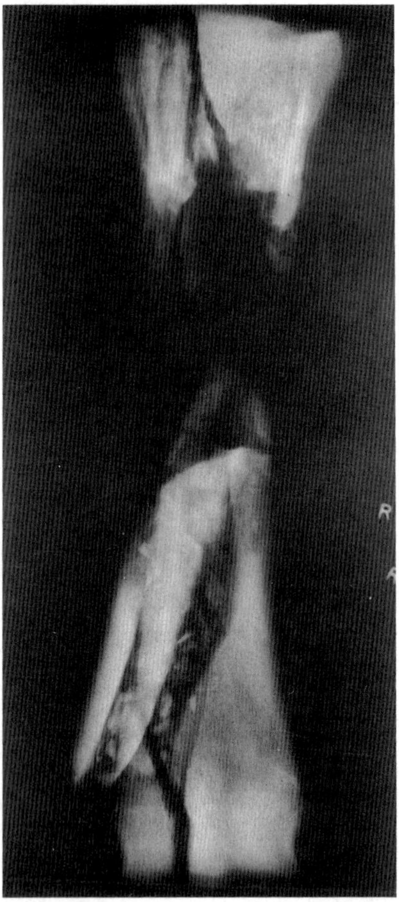

Fig. 117. A 3-year-old thoroughbred filly that fractured the right cannon bone. Both ends are involved, and the shaft is shattered. The fracture is comminuted and compound. Several pieces of the shaft are missing. The relationship between the parts of the cannon bone as it was after the fracture has been maintained by leaving the flexor tendons and the suspensory ligament on the specimen.

keeping the flexor tendons and the suspensory ligament on the specimen. Upon gross examination the joint cartilages showed no remarkable changes other than the fractures. In a microscopic section of the lower end of the cannon bone parallel to the fracture (Fig. 118), the subchondral bone plate is very thick in the front end, and the thick bone bars (trabeculae) are projected vertically in relation to the bone plate. Toward the lowest point of the cannon bone, the bone plate becomes very thin and continues so through the entire back aspect. The

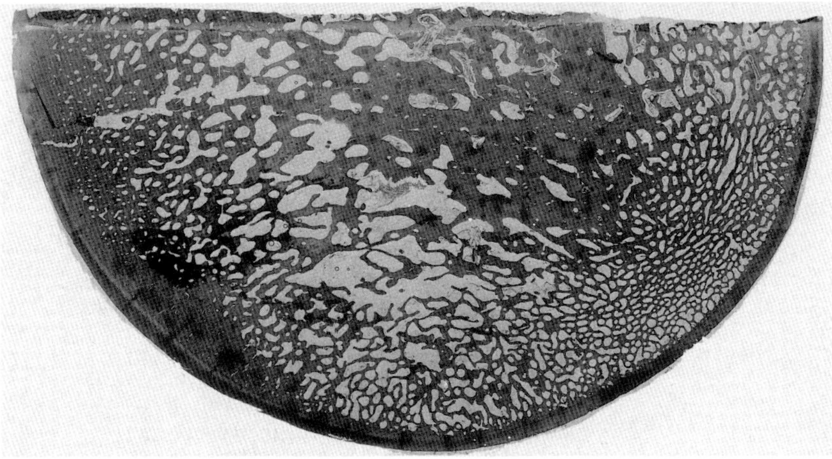

Fig. 118. Same horse as in Fig. 117. This microscopic section is through the inner condyle of the lower end of the right cannon bone parallel to the fracture. The front end is to the left. The subchondral bone plate of the front end is very thick, and so are the vertically arranged bone bars. The plate then becomes very narrow at the lowest and back parts. The bone bars in these areas are thin and arranged transversely. In the top right corner is a large area of osteopetrosis. ×2.7.

underlying trabeculae are thin and arranged transversely. These expressions of OCH constitute a weak point that, in our interpretation, causes the fracture.

These three first cases of cannon bone fractures have common denominators. All are caused by OCH. All cases have grossly normal joint cartilages. The changes described by radiography of slab section and by microscopy would not by themselves have caused clinical signs of lameness. A clinical radiographical examination would not have uncovered the changes and, in absence of lameness, there would have been no reason for taking radiographs. The stress of racing may have triggered the fractures but did not cause them. The fractures are pathological without previous clinical signs, so that though the horses seem to be racing sound, the jockeys are riding a time bomb.

The next case is a 5-year-old thoroughbred stallion that fractured the lower end of the left cannon bone. We see in Fig. 119 that the fracture started through a large OCH change in the outer condyle.

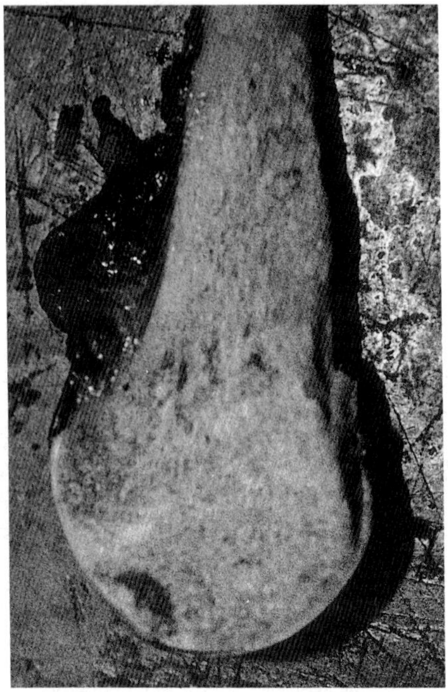

Fig. 119. A 5-year-old thoroughbred stallion that fractured the lower end of the left cannon bone. The fracture starts at the lower end of the outer condyle through a large OCH defect and extends obliquely upward to end in the shaft about 3 inches from the lower end.

The fracture went upward and ended some three inches into the outer part of the shaft. The flexor tendon of the left side was shown in Fig. 73 as an example of very severe mineralization. The horse thus showed severe OCH in the lower end of the cannon bone and very severe degeneration with mineralization of the flexor tendons. These changes together resulted in the fracture.

In Fig. 120 is the lower end of the right cannon one of a 3-year-old thoroughbred colt. The fracture concerned the outer condyle and went upward to include the lower end of the shaft. The fracture started through a severe OCH, and the rest of the lower end of the cannon bone also exhibited OCH, both of the inner condyle and of the ridge between the condyles. The lower end of the left cannon bone, which did not fracture, is shown in Fig. 121. There are extensive changes of OCD, the cartilage flaps are about to detach. In the sesamoid bones facing the fractured lower end of the right cannon bone, there is vast destruction of the joint cartilage (Fig. 122). There can be no doubt that the fracture occurred because of extensive OCH. One wonders how this horse ever made it to the starting gate.

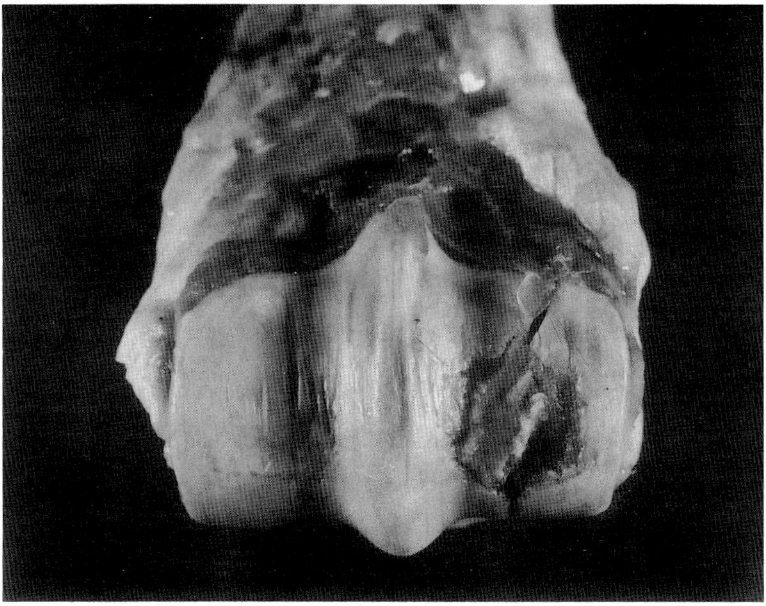

Fig. 120. A 3-year-old thoroughbred colt that fractured the lower end of the right cannon bone. The picture shows the lower end of the right cannon bone, from behind. There is a fracture beginning in the outer condyle through an area of severe OCH. The inner condyle (left) and the ridge between the condyles present numerous and deep grooves in the cartilage.

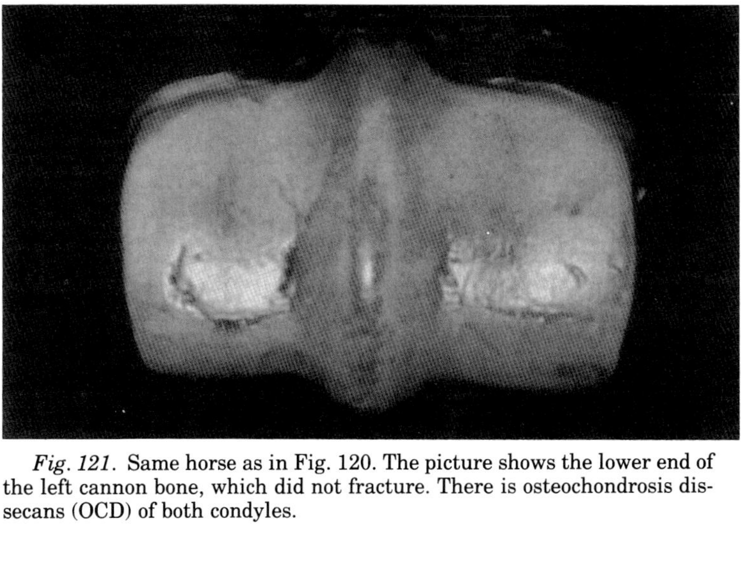

Fig. 121. Same horse as in Fig. 120. The picture shows the lower end of the left cannon bone, which did not fracture. There is osteochondrosis dissecans (OCD) of both condyles.

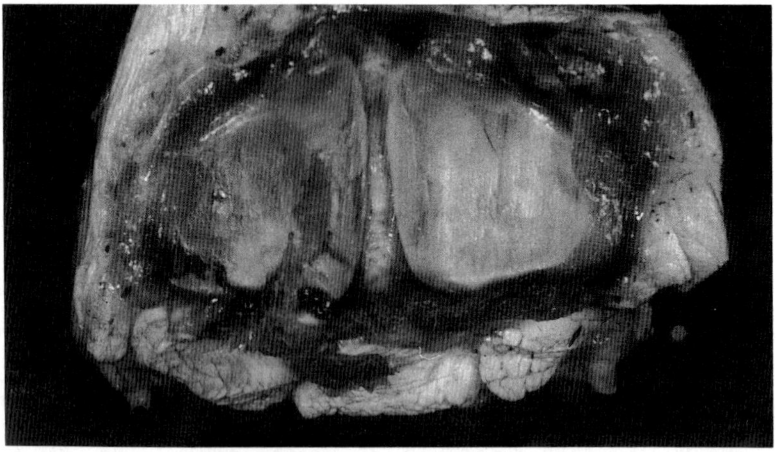

Fig. 122. Same horse as in Fig. 120 showing the sesamoid bones facing the lower end of the right cannon bone. There is vast destruction of the cartilage.

The fracture in the last-mentioned case is referred to as a Salter IV fracture. The typical radiographic picture in Fig. 123 shows a 10-year-old thoroughbred gelding.

All cases of fractures involving either or both ends of the cannon bone showed OCH as the underlying cause. In cases of shaft fractures without involvement of either end, OCH was not present and should not be expected. In these cases, tendon degeneration was commonly recorded. We see in Fig. 124 a dramatic illustration of this point. A 4-year-old thoroughbred colt fractured the left cannon bone. The fracture was comminuted and compound (Fig. 124a). No changes were found by radiography and microscopy in the bone tissue to explain the fracture. The left deep flexor tendon showed a hemorrhagic necrosis. It started just above the level of the sasamoid bones and continued about six inches upward (Figs. 124b,c,d). Seen from the surface that faces the superficial flexor tendon, the piece (c) is shown in Fig. 124e. There are two needle marks. The picture of the tendon cut crosswise through these needle marks are shown in Figs. 124f,g. The path of the needle describes a localized hemorrhage that leads into the central and extensive hemorrhagic necrosis.

The tendon damage is this case is acute, and the resulting fracture of the cannon bone must have happened within a short period of time after the tendon injections. No information about the injections was available, because such treatments are closely guarded secrets.

Chronic tendon damage was more common in cases of cannon bone fractures which involved the shaft only. One example is shown in Fig. 71. The left deep flexor tendon is from 4-year-old thoroughbred filly which fractured her left cannon bone, shaft only. The picture shows extensive tendon necrosis with heavy mineral deposits.

Figs. 74 and 75 show the left deep flexor tendon of a 5-year-old thoroughbred gelding which fractured his left cannon bone. The pictures show severe chronic tendon degeneration.

In summary, fractures of the cannon bone are, in the cases presented here, pathological, caused by OCH of either end or by tendon degeneration in cases of fractures of the shaft.

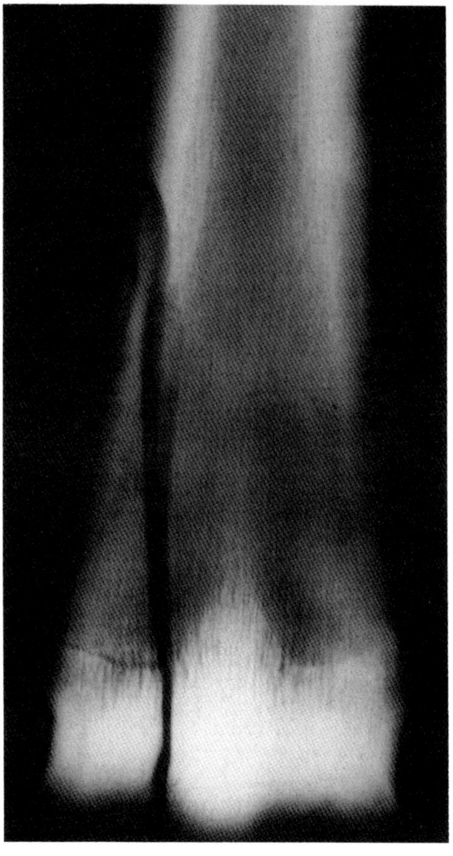

Fig. 123. The radiograph shows a fracture through the outer condyle of a 10-year-old thoroughbred gelding that fractured the right cannon bone. There is another fracture transversely just above the epiphysis, the dense white area, of the right condyle.

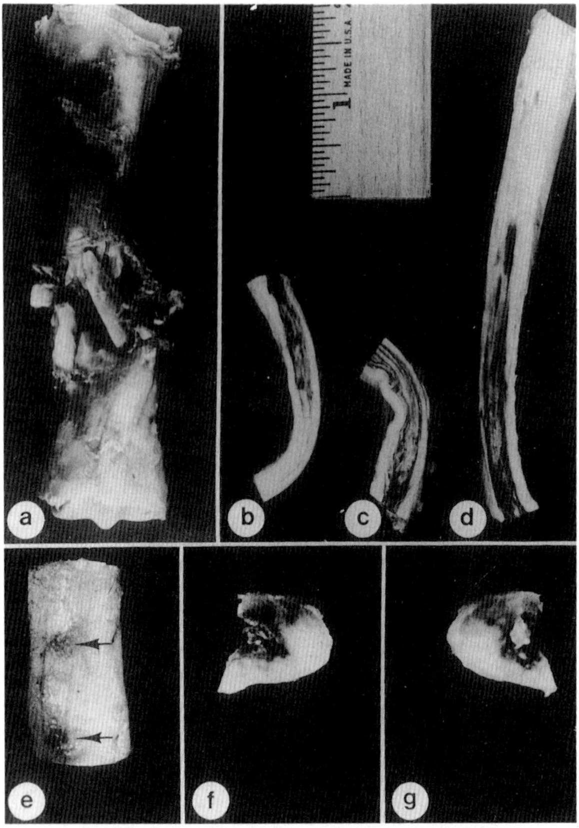

Fig. 124. A 4-year-old thoroughbred colt that fractured the left cannon bone. a shows a comminuted fracture of the left cannon bone; b, c and d are lengthwise sections through the deep flexor tendon of the left front limb. b starts just above the level of the sesamoid bones. The dark areas within the tendon represent a hemorrhagic necrosis. About 6 inches of the tendon shows this change (b + c + d).

e is the outer side of the part of the deep flexor tendon shown in c. In front of the arrows are needle marks. f is a transverse section through the area at the upper arrow in c. At the entrance into the tendon are hemorrhages which extend deep into the tendon. g is a similar section through the area of the lower arrow in e. Same thing as in f.

E. *The sesamoid bones*

There were 19 cases: 2 colts, 3 fillies, 8 geldings, 5 stallions and 1 mare. The ages of the horses were: 2 3-year-olds, 6 4-year-olds, 7 5-year-olds, 2 6-year-olds, and 2 7-year-olds. In 7 cases, one sesamoid bone was fractured and in 12 cases both sesamoid bones of the same side were fractured. There were 16 transverse fractures and 15 were comminuted. The upper end was fractured in 2 cases, the middle portion in 23, and the lower end in 6 cases. OCH was observed in 8 cases and CON in 10 cases. The changes were not so severe as to be interpreted as the primary cause of the fractures. The flexor tendons and the suspensory ligament were examined in 17 of the 19 cases, and all showed tendon degeneration as illustrated in Figs. 69-81 in the beginning of this chapter.

A 4-year-old thoroughbred gelding fractured the inner sesamoid bone of the left front limb (Fig. 125). The capsule of the fetlock joint, both branches of the suspensory ligament and both flexor tendons were ruptured. The cannon bone was completely separated from the sesamoid bones and from the long pastern bone. The periosteum (the bone membrane) was stripped from the lower two thirds of the cannon bone.

In the next case, a 5-year-old thoroughbred gelding fractured both left sesamoid bones (Fig. 126). There is ample evidence of OCH at the upper end of the sesamoid bones, but the OCH changes are not associated with the fractures. The inner branch of the suspensory ligament is ruptured.

Another 5-year-old thoroughbred gelding fractured the inner left sesamoid bone (Fig. 127). There are, again, OCH changes at the top of all 4 sesamoid bones, but the changes are not associated with the fracture. The lower sesamoidean ligaments, which run from the lower ends of the sesamoid bones to the back side of the long pastern bone, are shredded almost beyond recognition. Both branches of the suspensory ligament and the deep flexor tendon showed chronic degeneration. The changes in the other bones of the fetlock joint were severe and revealing (Figs. 128-130). The lower ends of the cannon bones are seen from front in Fig. 128. The CON changes are extreme, with vast destruction of cartilage and bone. The back aspect of the lower ends of the cannon bones (Fig. 129) are equally affected with deep cracks in and detachment of cartilage. The upper ends of the long pastern bones show equally extensive damage by CON (Fig. 130).

With severe degeneration of the flexor tendon and the branches of the suspensory ligament, with OCH of the sesamoid bones and severe CON changes in the cannon bone and the long pastern bone, it is easy to understand why a fracture occurred. What is not so easy to understand is how this horse ever made it to the starting gate. The horse could not possibly have been racing sound with all these documented changes. The only way to get a horse with such fetlock joints to the

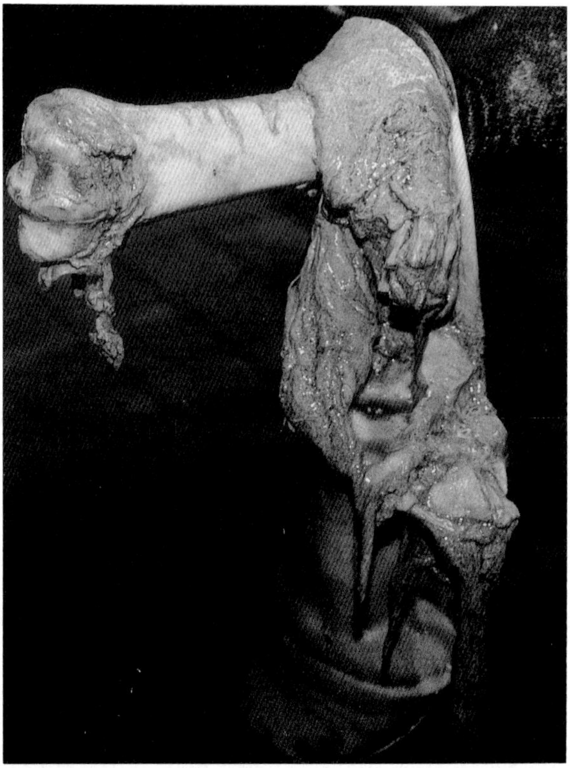

Fig. 125. A 4-year-old thoroughbred gelding that fractured the inner left sesamoid bone. The knee is at top; the specimen is viewed from front. The inner sesamoid bone is fractured (center right in the picture). The entire fetlock joint is disrupted because all ligaments and tendons have ruptured. The cannon bone, which points to the left in the upper part, has its bone membrane (periosteum) detached well beyond the midshaft.

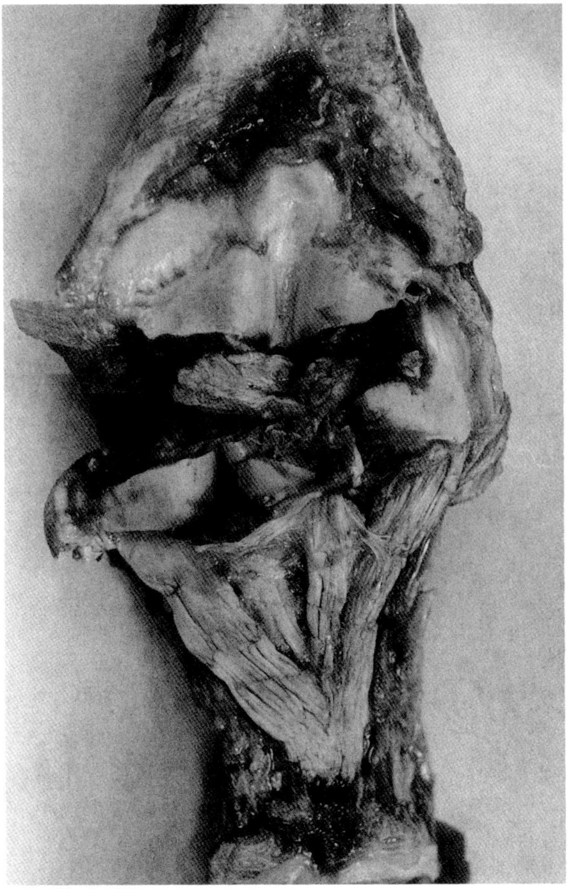

Fig. 126. A 5-year-old thoroughbred stallion that fractured both sesamoid bones of the left front limb. Both fractures are comminuted. The inner branch of the suspensory ligament (to the left) is torn. The upper ends of the sesamoid bones present OCH changes, but the fractures do not occur within such changes.

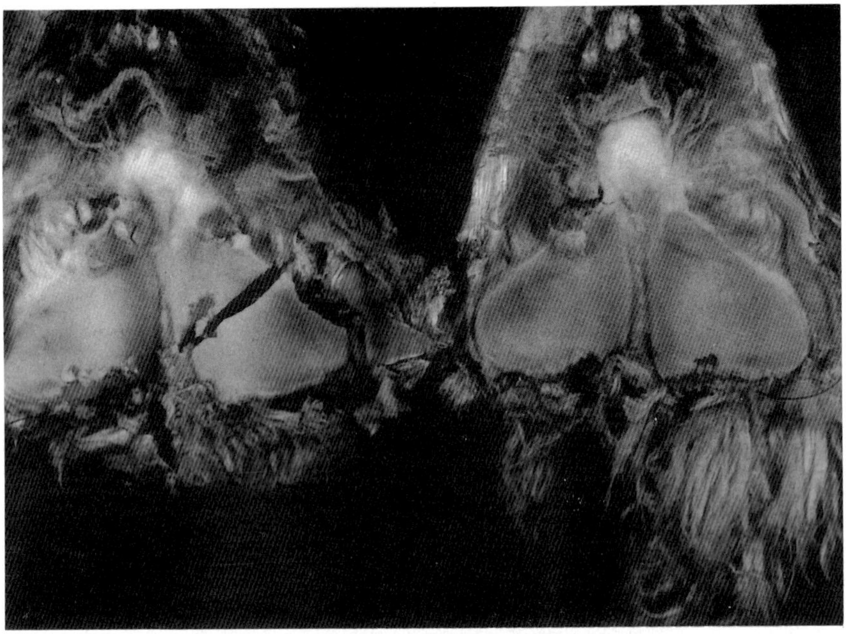

Fig. 127. A 5-year-old thoroughbred gelding that fractured the inner sesamoid bone of the left front limb. The sesamoid bones are viewed from the front. There is severe OCH at the upper part of all four sesamoid bones. There is a transverse fracture of the inner left sesamoid bone. The fracture is not associated with OCH changes. The ligaments at the lower end of the sesamoid bones are torn.

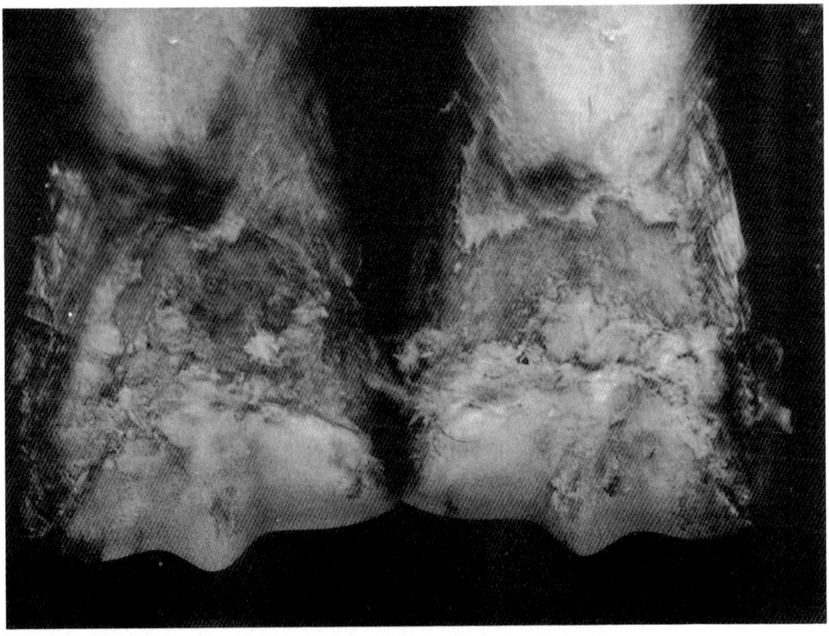

Fig. 128. Same horse as in Fig. 127. The pictures show the lower end of the cannon bones seen from front. There are severe and extensive CON changes.

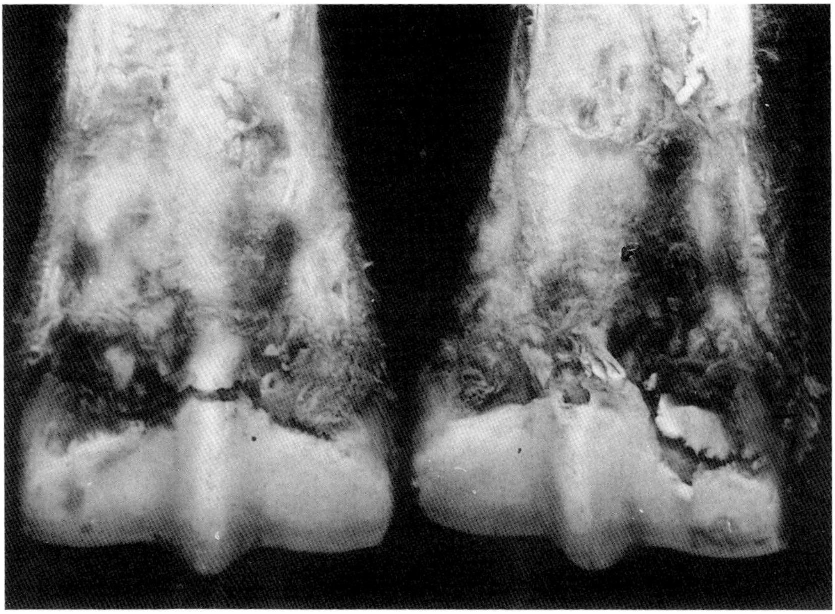

Fig. 129. Same horse as in Fig. 128. The pictures show the lower end of the cannon bone seen from behind. There are very severe CON change. The ridge between the condyles is separated and so is a large piece of cartilage of the medial condyle (to the right).

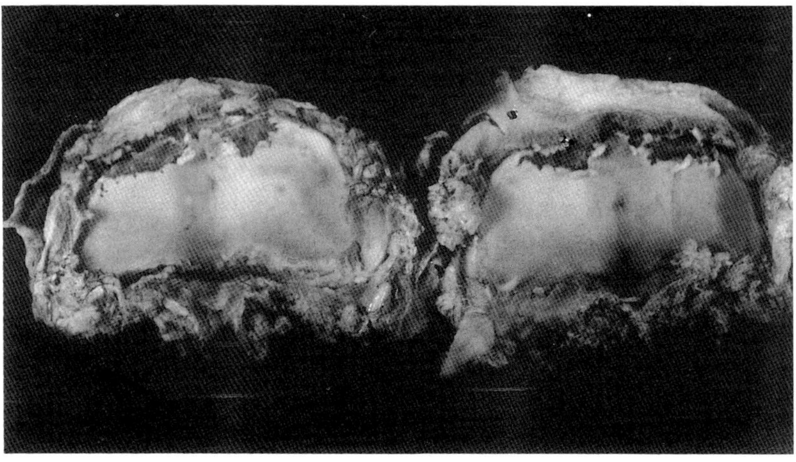

Fig. 130. Same horse as in Fig. 128. The long pastern bones are seen from above. There is severe CON of the front end (top) and, to a lesser degree, of the back end.

starting gate is, we believe, to extinguish the clinical signs by injections into the joint with a pain-killing agent. The CON lesions indicate that this had happened repeatedly.

As stated above, sesamoid bone fractures occurred with degeneration of tendons and ligaments in all cases examined microscopically. We will now add two more cases with illustration of both. A 3-year-old thoroughbred gelding fractured both left sesamoid bones (Fig. 131). Both branches of the suspensory ligament are torn. The microscopic changes in these branches are illustrated in Figs. 72, 76, and 77. The damage to these structures is extensive and chronic and certainly explains the fracture of the sesamoid bones.

An equally dramatic case is presented in Fig. 132. A 5-year-old thoroughbred gelding fractured both left front limb sesamoid bones. The microscopic changes of the deep flexor tendon of that bone appear in Figs. 78-80. There is virtually no tendon tissue left, and the replacing scar tissue shows prominent formation of bone tissue. Such a tendon has lost all its elasticity, and the pathologic mechanical forces therefore transmitted to the sesamoid bones caused the fracture. Again, if we look at bones as a functional unit which also includes the tendons, the fractures are pathological.

F. *The long pastern bone*

There were two cases: 1 in a 4-year-old colt and 1 in a 5-year-old stallion.

The upper end of the left long pastern bone of the first case is shown in Fig. 133. The comminuted fracture split the upper end in the midline and shattered the inner part into several pieces. There were OCH changes at the upper front end, and the fracture ran through these changes. The radiograph (Fig. 134) in front view showed that the fracture involved both ends and that the body was shattered. There were two transverse screws in the lower end of the cannon bone, supposedly from a previously treated case of a Salter IV fracture. A microscopic section parallel to one of the fracture lines of the inner part of the upper end presented a roller-coaster contour with dales leaving the underlying bone exposed and the hills quite shallow (Fig. 135). The cartilage was pale, and there was minimal differentiation of cells. There was no zone of calcified cartilage and no bone plate beneath the joint cartilage. All trabeculae were arranged transversely.

In the second case (Fig. 136), the shattering of the upper end of the right front long pastern bone was so severe that an evaluation of the joint cartilage was not possible. The radiograph (Fig. 137) from inside-outside showed vast destruction of the upper end, as well as a comminuted fracture of the body of the long pastern bone. The radiograph did not show conclusively the involvement of the lower end, but a gross picture did (Fig. 138). The lower end of the adjoining cannon bone (Fig. 139) showed severe CON changes.

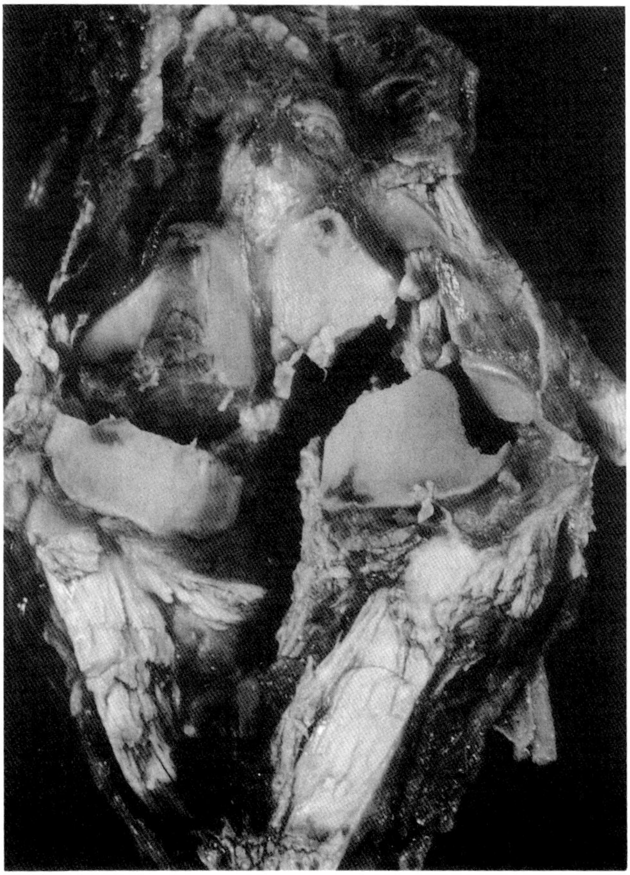

Fig. 131. A 3-year-old thoroughbred gelding that fractured both sesamoid bones of the left front limb. There are comminuted fractures of both bones. Both branches of the suspensory ligament and the lower sesamoid ligament are ruptured and shredded.

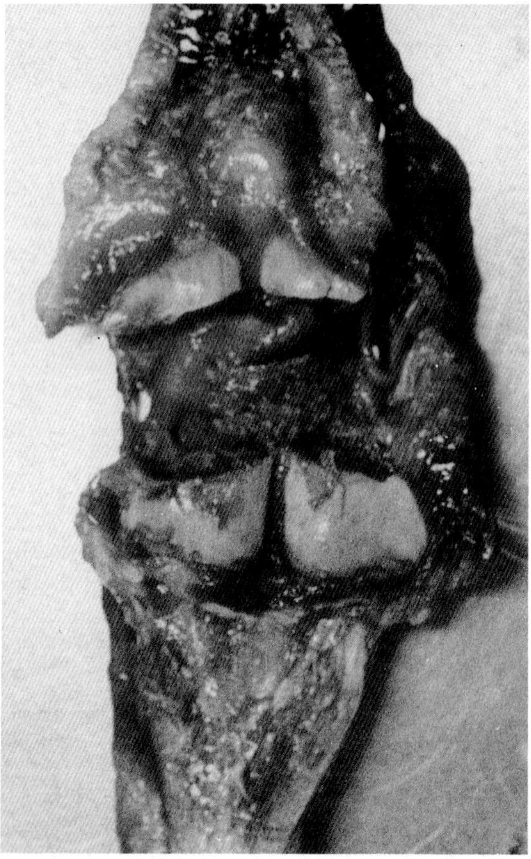

Fig. 132. A 5-year-old thoroughbred gelding that fractured both sesamoid bones of the left front limb. There are transverse fractures of both bones Both branches of the suspensory ligaments are ruptured.

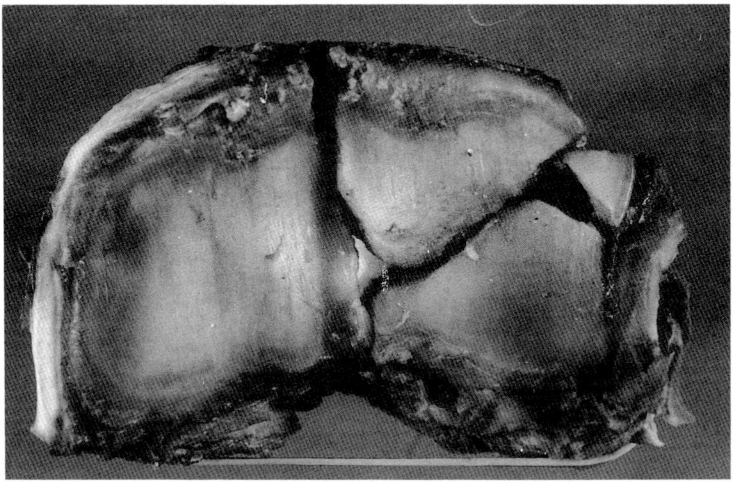

Fig. 133. A 4-year-old thoroughbred colt with a fracture of the left long pastern bone. Viewed from above there is a comminuted fracture. The front end presents moderate OCH changes.

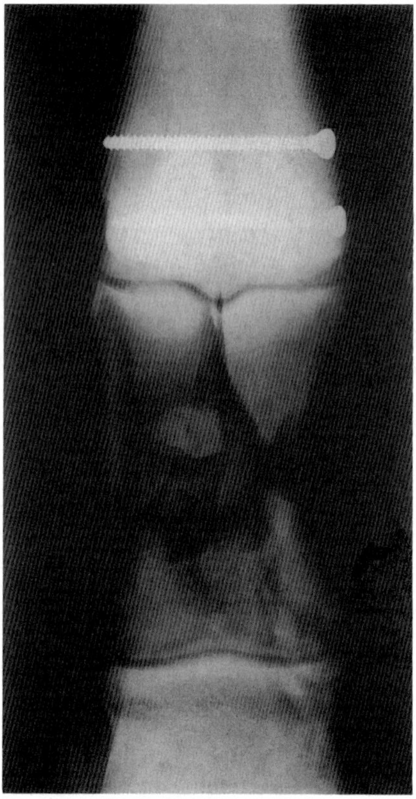

Fig. 134. Same horse as in Fig. 133. Radiograph from front of the long pastern bone. The fracture involves the upper end, shatters the body, and goes down through the lower end. There is a screw in the lower end of the cannon bone, a surgically treated fracture of that end.

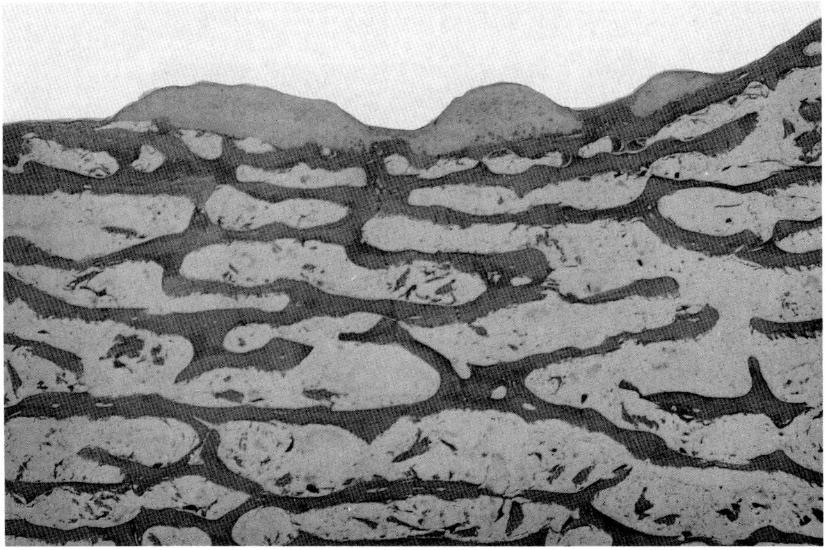

Fig. 135. Same horse as in Fig. 133. This is a microscopic section through the upper end of the long pastern bone of the left side. The contour of the joint cartilage is that of a roller-coaster. To the far left and right there is no cartilage cover of the trabeculae, which are uniformly thin and arranged transversely. ×14.

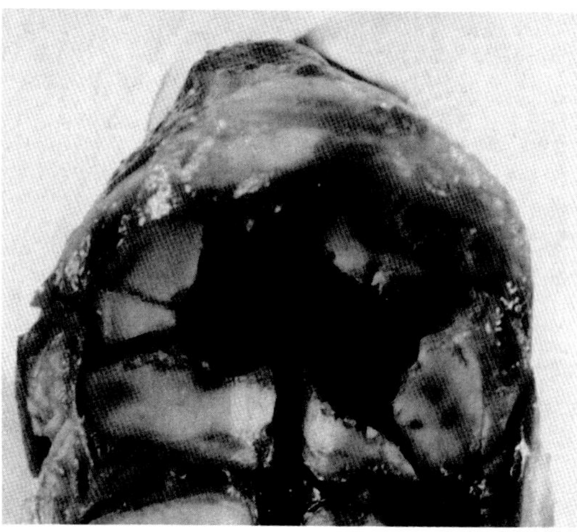

Fig. 136. A 5-year-old thoroughbred stallion that fractured the right long pastern bone. There is a comminuted fracture, with many of the bone fragments lost.

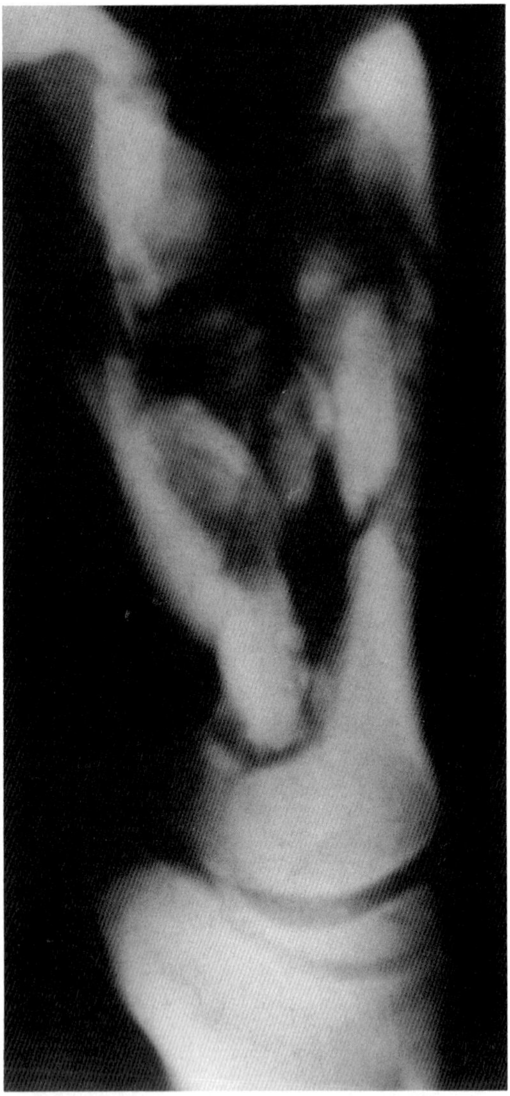

Fig. 137. Same horse as in Fig. 136. Radiograph from inside of the right front long pastern bone. There is a comminuted fracture, with many of the bone fragments lost.

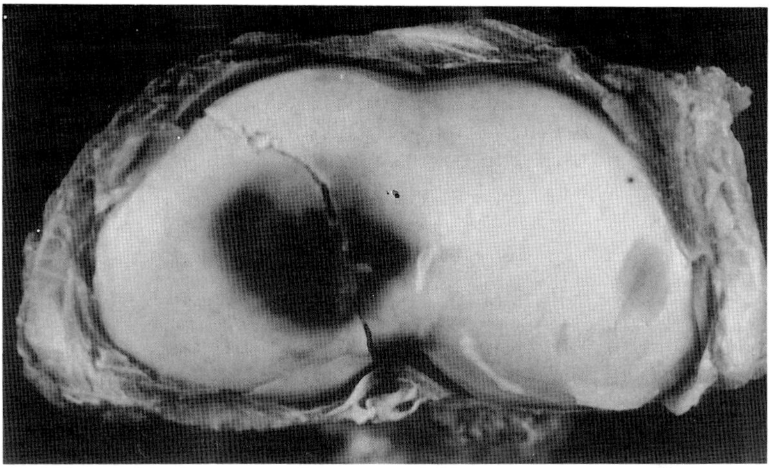

Fig. 138. Same horse as in Fig. 136. The pictures show the lower end of the right front long pastern bone. A fracture line extends obliquely through the outer condyle. The dark area is bloodstained cartilage. Note that this fracture did not show in the radiograph in Fig. 137.

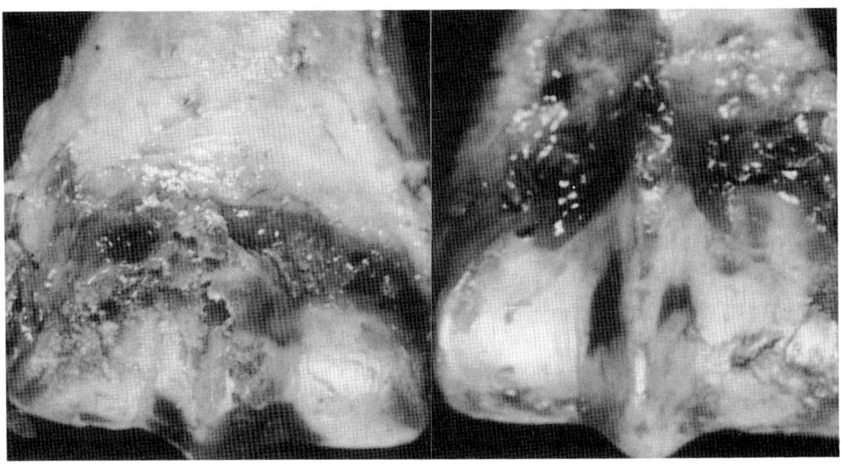

Fig. 139. Same horse as in Fig. 136. The picture shows the lower end of the right front cannon bone viewed from front (left) and behind (right). There is very severe CON. Note especially the advanced damage of the cartilage and bone at the upper part of the end viewed from front.

Microscopic examination of several pieces of the shattered upper end of the long pastern bone showed severe changes of the joint cartilage as described above.

The first case is unquestionably one of OCH. All microscopic changes documented meet our definition of OCH: failure of cartilage to convert into bone. The pre-existing evidence of a Salter IV fracture lends further support for this view.

In the second case, the gross changes of the fractured long pastern bone were so severe that a sampling for microscopic examination may not have been adequate. The changes documented strongly suggested corticosteroid exposure. Further, and most importantly, the adjoining cannon bone showed severe CON. We have never observed these changes in one bone of a joint without involvement of the other. The co-existent changes in the cannon bone and the long pastern bone are, we believe, strong evidence for injections of corticosteroids into the fetlock joint.

G. *The coffin bone*

There was 1 case: A 3-year-old gelding fractured the right front coffin bone.

This fracture occurred at some unknown time before submission to necropsy. The fracture extended from the joint cartilage to the lower end of the bone and concerned the outer part (Fig. 140). On microscopic examination, the separated bone surfaces were joined by a callus, too old to give any information on why the fracture occured.

H. *The tibia*

There was 1 case: A 3-year-old filly fractured the right tibia.

The fracture occurred within one furlong after the start. The fracture involved the upper end and was comminuted as shown in Fig. 141, in which the displaced parts were tied together. The inner condyle is very short in the radiograph exposed from in front. Instead of going upward to form the spine of the tibia, the inner condyle ends abruptly, dips down, and forms a large concavity. One of the many fracture lines begins at the lowest part of this concavity and goes down into an area of severely shattered bone. A radiograph of a slab section from outside to inside of this part (Fig. 142) shows that the contour of the upper end of the condyle is horizontal to the right and middle of the picture but then dips abruptly into a deep concavity to the left, where the spine should have projected upward. Note that there is osteopetrosis inside this concavity. A fracture line starts at the lowest point of the concavity. In the next picture, Fig. 143, we see the *normal* picture of a comparable radiograph of a slab section. Please note the height of the spine.

Next we present a microscopic section through the spine of the tibia cut from inside (right) to toward the middle (left) of the upper end of the right tibia (Fig. 144). The picture and its legend show that we are dealing with OCH.

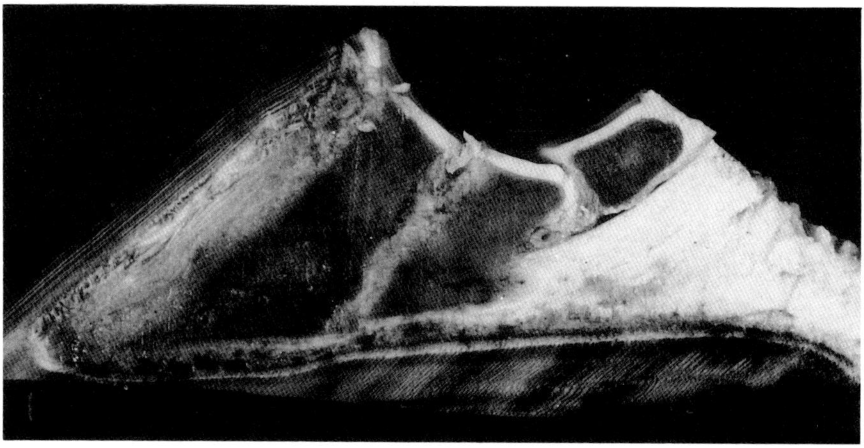

Fig. 140. A 3-year-old thoroughbred gelding that fractured the right front coffin bone. The fracture extends from the joint cartilage to the lower end of the bone. The callus is thick.

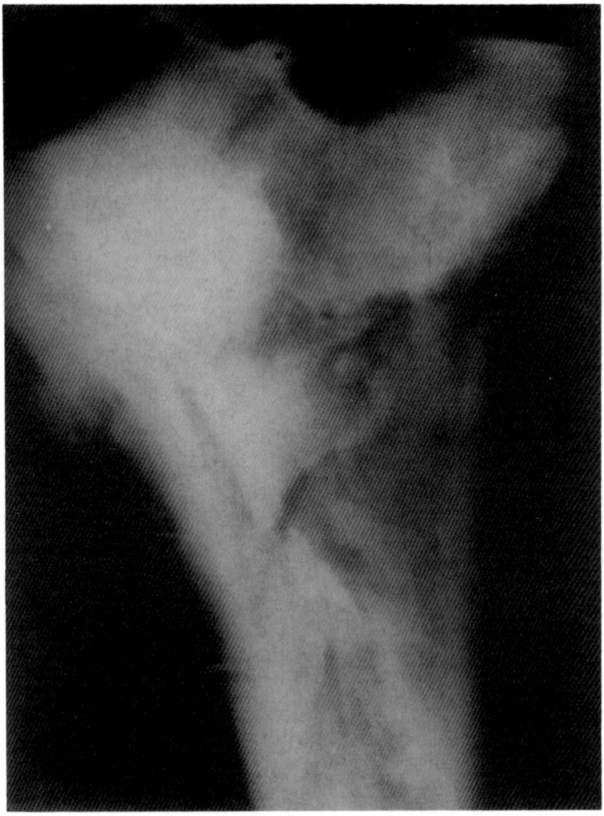

Fig. 141. A 3-year-old thoroughbred filly that fractured her right tibia. The radiograph is taken from front; inside is to the right. The shattered pieces have been tied together.

There is a comminuted fracture with many fracture lines. The spine of the tibia is very shallow. The inner condyle ends abruptly to form a deep concavity rather than to extend upward to form the spine.

Note that a fracture line starts at the lowest point of the concavity and goes straight downward.

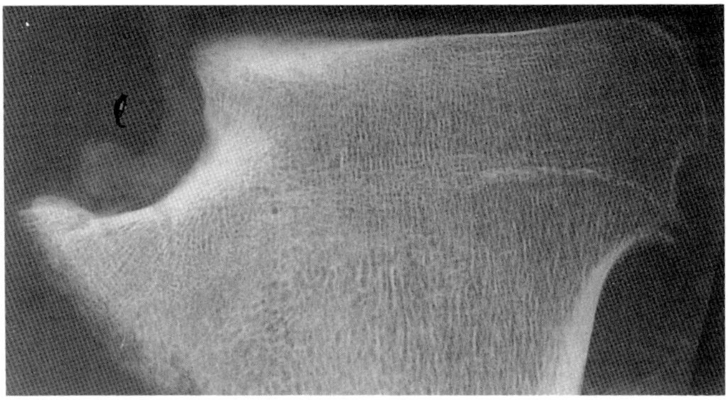

Fig. 142. Same filly as in Fig. 141. The radiograph shows a slab section of the inner condyle cut from inside (right) toward the middle. The contour of the upper end of the condyle is horizontal to the right and middle of the picture, but then dips abruptly into a deep concavity to the left, where the spine should have projected upward. There is osteopetrosis inside the concavity. A fracture line starts at the lowest point of the concavity.

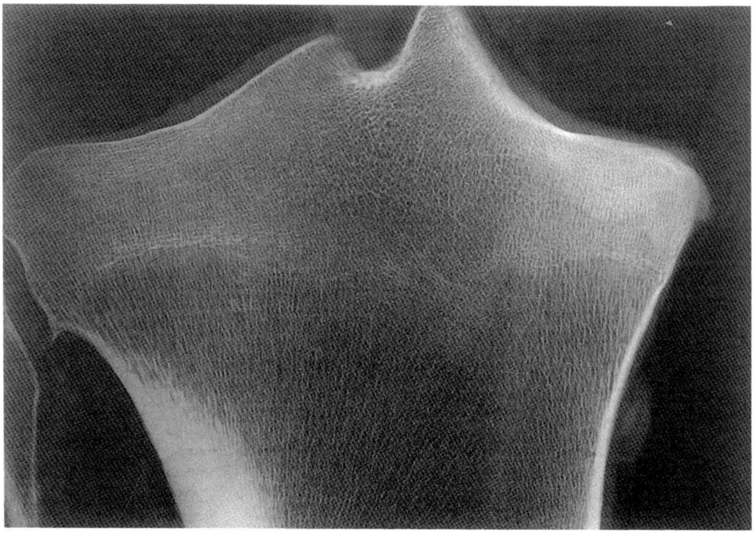

Fig. 143. A 4-year-old thoroughbred gelding that fractured the right shoulder blade. The picture shows the radiograph of a slab section through the right tibia oriented as in Fig. 142. This is a *normal* architecture. Note the height of the spine of the tibia.

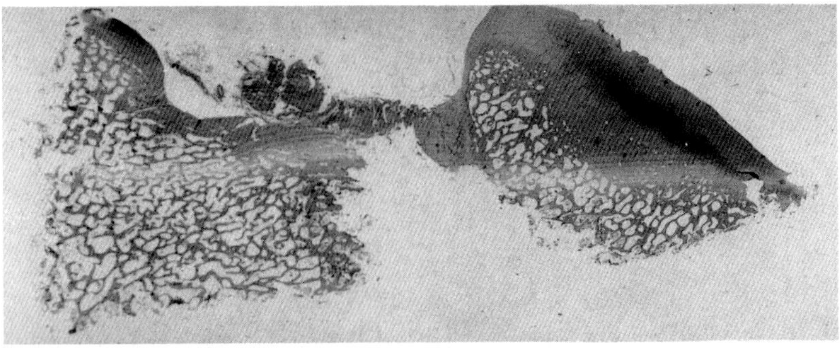

Fig. 144. Same filly as in Fig. 141. The microscopic picture shows a section from inside (right) toward the middle and part of the outside condyle (left) of the upper end of the right tibia. The cartilage to the far right is deeply stained, and there is pronounced petrosis of the underlying bone. Going to the left, the cartilage loses its normal deep staining, and then stops abruptly. Instead of presenting a rising spine, the contour dips into a deep concavity at the bottom of which the cruciate ligaments are attached. The outside condyle to the far left is also not producing the spine. The cone-shaped gap in the lower right center is a fracture. ×1.7.

I. *The coffin bone (hind limb)*

There was one case: A 5-year-old stallion which fractured the coffin bone of the right hind limb.

The fracture involved the outer ¼, started at the joint cartilage, but did not reach the sole (Fig. 145). There were no microscopic changes in the bone to explain the fracture but the deep flexor tendon showed severe degeneration with mineral deposits and cartilage-forming cells (Fig. 81).

J. *The second loin vertebra*

There was one case: A 3-year-old filly.

Both hind limbs suddenly became paralyzed during a race. Post mortem examination revealed a fracture of the second loin vertebra (Fig. 146) with the third loin vertebra displaced downward and severe traumatization of the spinal cord. In this picture you see in the third vertebra (to the left of the fractured second vertebra) a thin white line near the lowest part of that bone. A similar but less-well-defined line is present in the second vertebra. The lines represent the last remnants of the cartilage which forms the ventral crest. Ventral denotes a position toward the belly, so the ventral part of a vertebra is the lower part. The upper part is referred to as dorsal. The ventral longitudinal ligament is attached to this crest; this ligament shows as the dense white band beneath the vertebrae in Fig. 146.

In the third loin vertebra, which did not fracture, we see in Fig. 147 the last remnants of the fetal cartilage. The bone above this carti-

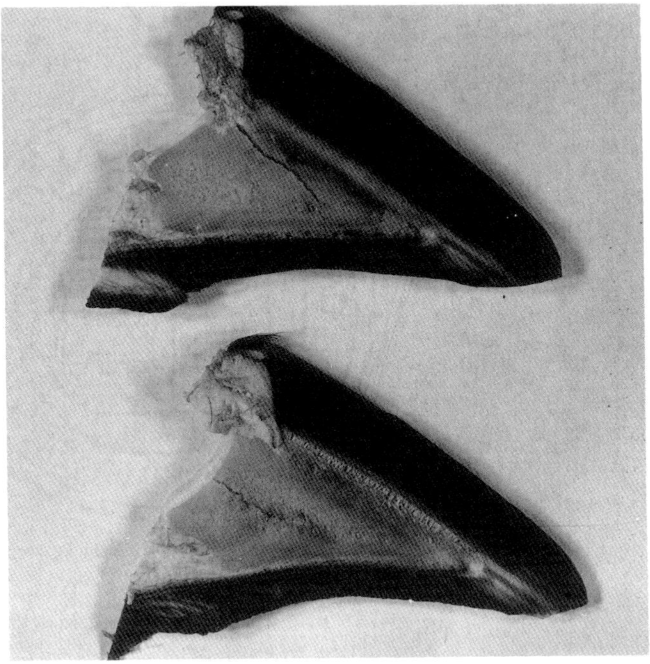

Fig. 145. A 5-year-old thoroughbred stallion that fractured the right hind coffin bone. The pictures are from sections outside the midline. In the top part, the fracture line extends from the joint cartilage toward the sole but does not reach it. In the lower part, the fracture line starts further out in the joint cartilage.

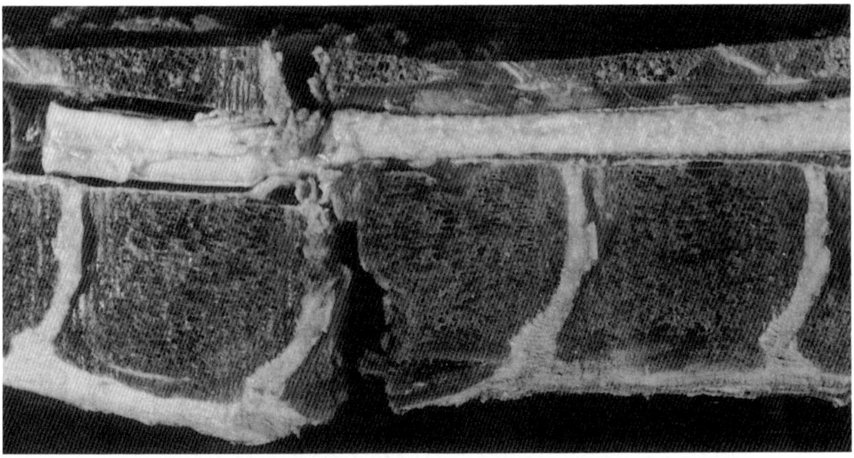

Fig. 146. A 3-year-old thoroughbred filly that fractured her 2nd loin back bone. The picture shows a length-wise section through the middle of the front part of the loin region. To the left is the most front part of the 4th loin bone, the 3rd, 2nd, and 1st loin bones; the back end of the last chest back bone is to the far right. The 2nd loin back bone is fractured at its back part. The 2nd loin back bone is displaced upward and the spinal cord is almost severed.

Note the white band inside the lower border of the 3rd loin back bone and, less well defined, on the lower border of the 2nd loin back bone.

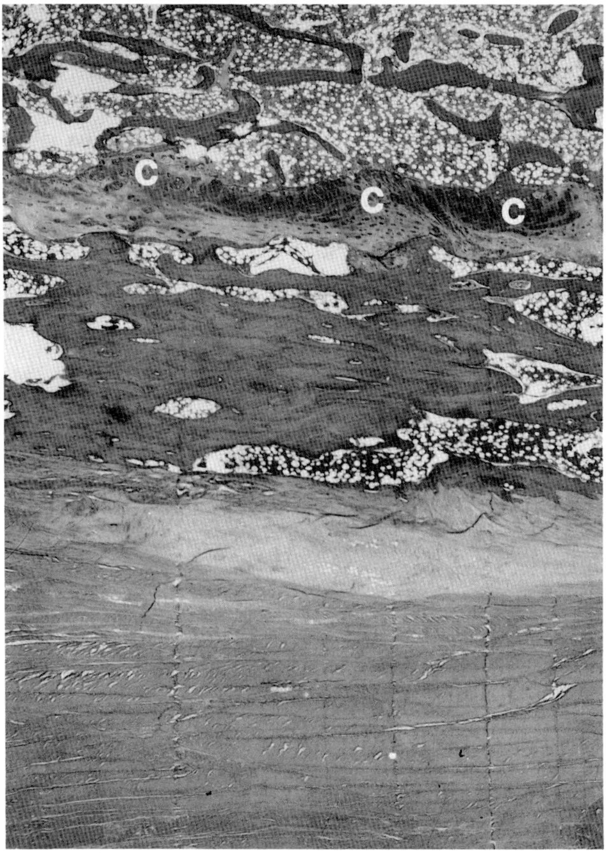

Fig. 147. Same filly as in Fig. 146. Microscopic section through the lower part of the 3rd loin back bone (which did not fracture). The horizontal band marked c corresponds to the white line in the gross specimen. The area marked c is the last remnant of the cartilage that forms the ventral crest. The bone above the cartilage consists of slender trabecular bone, the bone below the cartilage is dense. Beneath the crest is the ventral longitudinal ligament. ×12.

lage is trabecular, and the crest itself consists of dense bone. Beneath this dense bone is the ventral longitudinal ligament. Fig. 147 represents the normal picture of a vertebra approaching the final stage of growth.

Now back to the second vertebra. A radiograph of a midline slab section (Fig. 148) shows that the fracture detaches the ventral crest, then moves upwards to detach about ¾ of the back portion of the vertebra. A microscopic section through the ventral part is shown in Fig. 149. The fracture line goes between areas of retained cartilage. The separation within the retained cartilage must have been present before the fracture, as evidenced by Figs. 150 and 151. In these pictures, at higher magnification than in Fig. 149, the facing cartilages have been placed more closely together. All four cartilages show severe OCH changes. The cartilage is pale, the cells are few and arranged in no order. Significantly, the facing contours do not match at all. Equally significant is the finding that the lower piece of cartilage in Fig. 150 is lined at its top (which faces the gap) by a thin layer of bone.

As the fracture line turned upward (Fig. 148) it, again, went through areas of OCH (Fig. 152). These areas of retained cartilage with cysts formation occurred in the same position as that of the back growth plate, remnants of which also appear in Fig. 152.

The fracture of the second loin vertebra was, without doubt, caused by OCH with OCD. This case also underlines the necessity of microscopic examination, without which this case would have been diagnosed as a traumatic fracture. The cartilage changes are in all respects similar to those described in OCH and OCD in joint cartilages. The concept that the various manifestations of OCH are caused by pressure within the joints are microfractures (1,2) from repetitive trauma, cannot clearly be supported. Instead, the illustrated changes supports our definition of OCH: a failure of cartilage to convert into bone.

Here ends the description of fractures occurring during races. There can be only one conclusion from these numerous illustrations: the fractures are pathological, not traumatic. The stress of racing may be a triggering factor, but not a cause. To underscore this point, we will present another fracture case, although it did not occur during a race.

A 4-year-old thoroughbred colt fractured the cannon bone, a sesamoid bone and the long pastern bone of the right front limb during a *light* workout. The radiographs of the fractured bones are presented in Figs. 153-155. The fracture of the cannon bone was a Salter IV fracture that started in the outer condyle of the cannon bone and went up to the shaft (Fig. 153). The fractures of the sesamoid bone and of the long pastern bones were comminuted (Figs. 154 and 155).

The gross appearance of the fractured bones is documented in Figs. 156-158. In all fractured bones, which are part of the fetlock

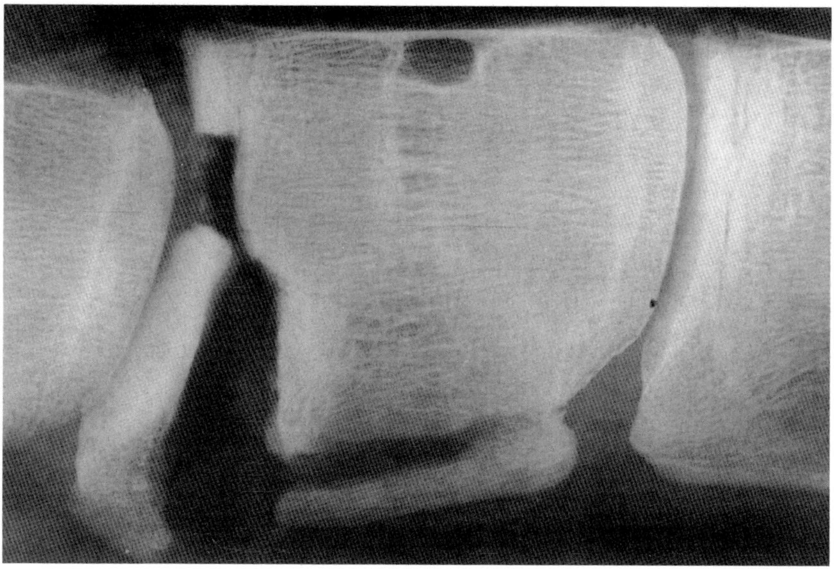

Fig. 148. Same filly as in Fig. 146. Radiograph shows a slab section with 2nd loin back bone in the center. The fracture detaches the ventral crest horizontally. The fracture line then runs upward to detach most of the back part of the bone. Note displacement of the 2nd or 3rd back bones.

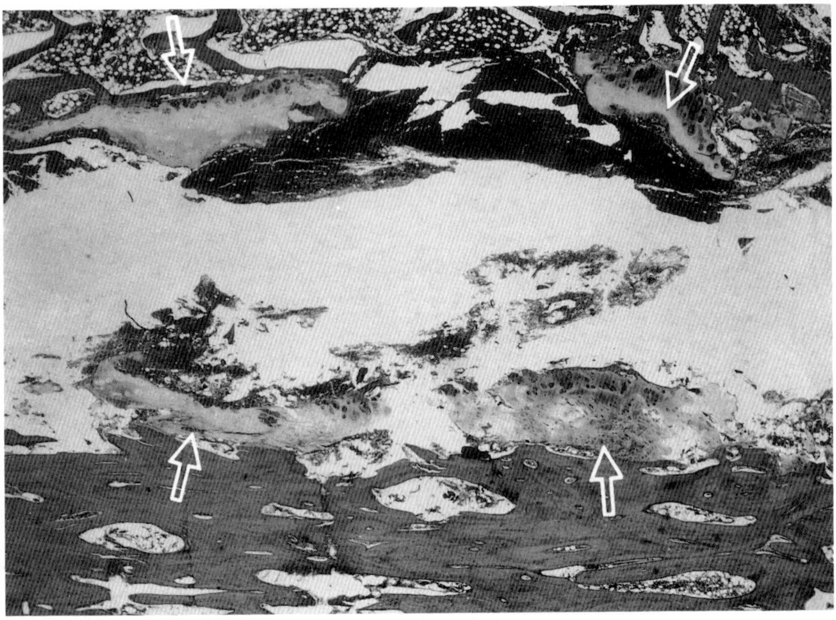

Fig. 149. Same filly as in Fig. 146. Microscopic section through the ventral part of the 2nd loin back bone. The ventral crest is at the lower part of the picture. The wide horizontal gap in the middle is the fracture site. In front of each arrow is a chunk of cartilage. The dark areas inside the cartilage is blood. $\times 12$.

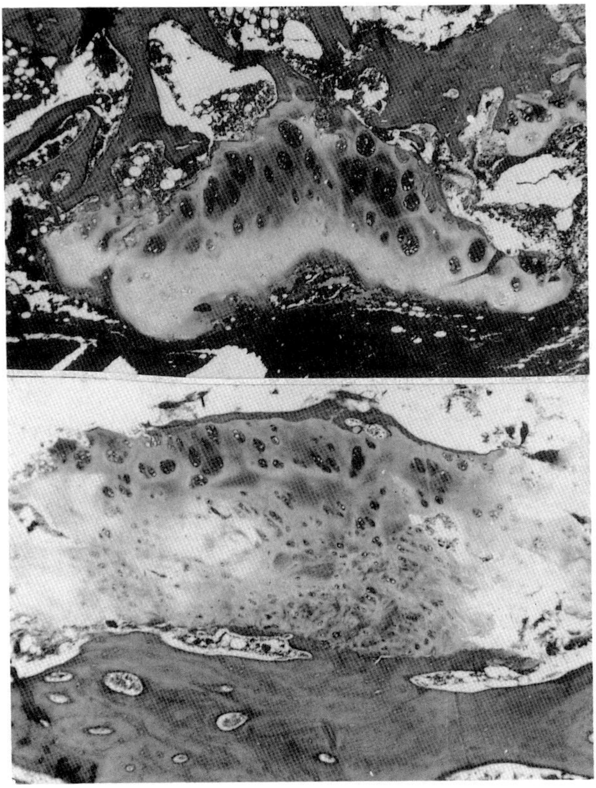

Fig. 150. Details of areas in front of right arrows in Fig. 149. The pictures of the upper and lower parts next to the fracture have been placed closer together than in Fig. 149. In the upper part, the cartilage facing the fracture is pale and has very few cells. The cartilage in the lower part, which sits on the ventral crest, shows poor and irregular staining, and the cartilage cells, which are few and of different sizes, show haphazard arrangement. The black line on top of that cartilage is bone tissue. The facing contours of the upper and lower cartilage pieces do not match at all. ×40.

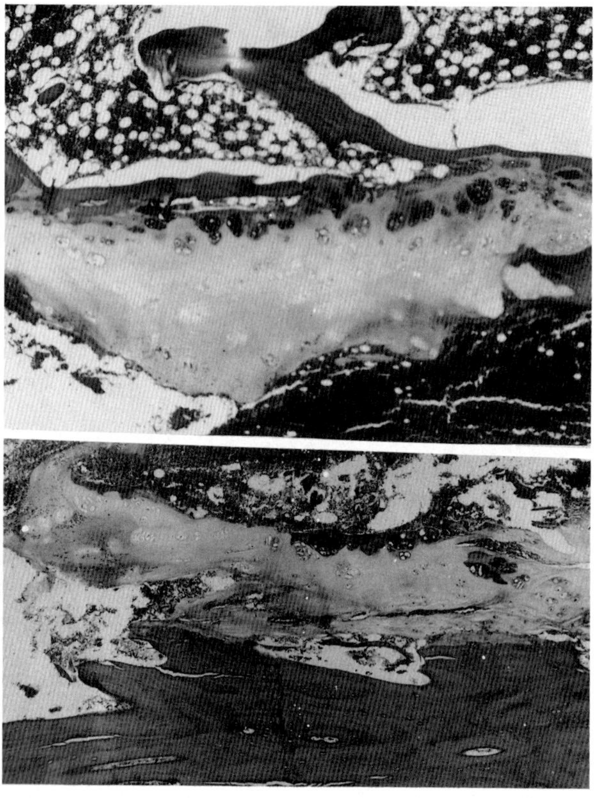

Fig. 151. Details of areas in front of the left arrows in Fig. 149. The upper and lower parts are arranged as in Fig. 150. In the upper part, there are a few cells at the top; otherwise the cartilage is very pale and almost without cells. The cartilage next to the ventral crest (lower part) is thin, pale, and has few cells. Again, the facing contours do not match at all. ×40.

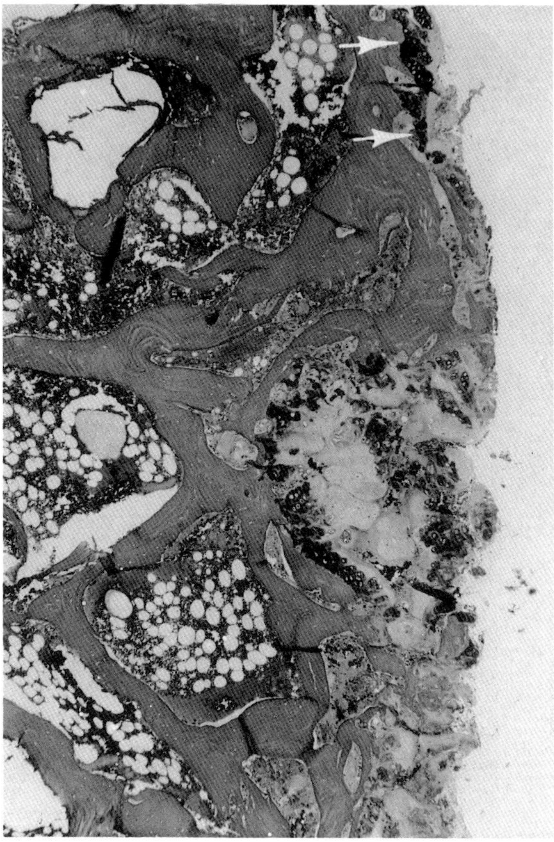

Fig. 152. This microscopic section is from the upper back end of the fracture shown in Figs. 146 and 148. The fracture line is to the right. In the middle part of the bone facing the fracture is a large area of cartilage. The cartilage is irregularly pale, and the cells are arranged in no particular order. Note that the fracture runs through this retained cartilage. In front of the arrows at top right is a thin layer of cartilage, presumably the remnants of the growth plate. ×45.

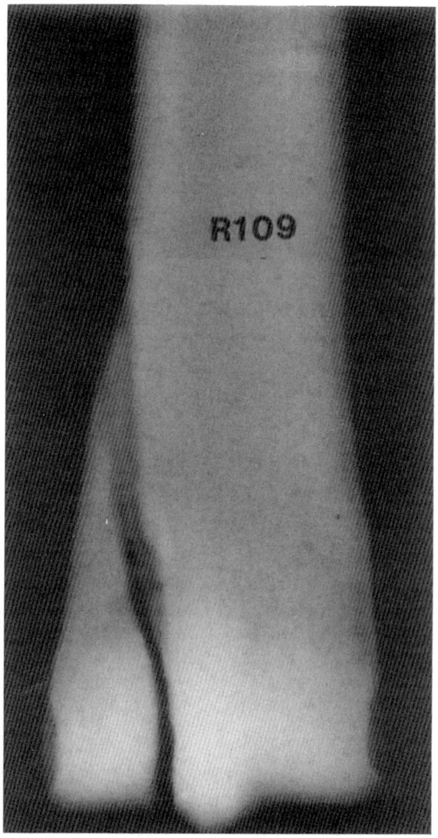

Fig. 153. This is a radiograph of the right front cannon bone, seen from front of a 4-year-old thoroughbred colt. The fracture starts in the outer condyle and goes up to the cortex (Salter IV fracture).

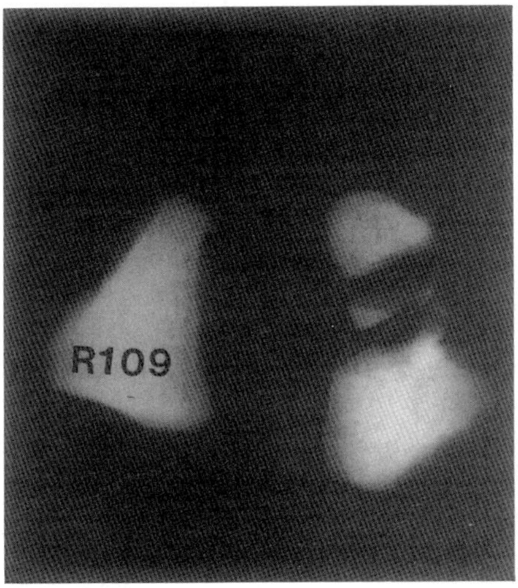

Fig. 154. Same horse as in Fig. 153. This is a radiograph of the sesamoid bones, right front limb seen from front. There is a comminuted fracture of the inner sesamoid bones.

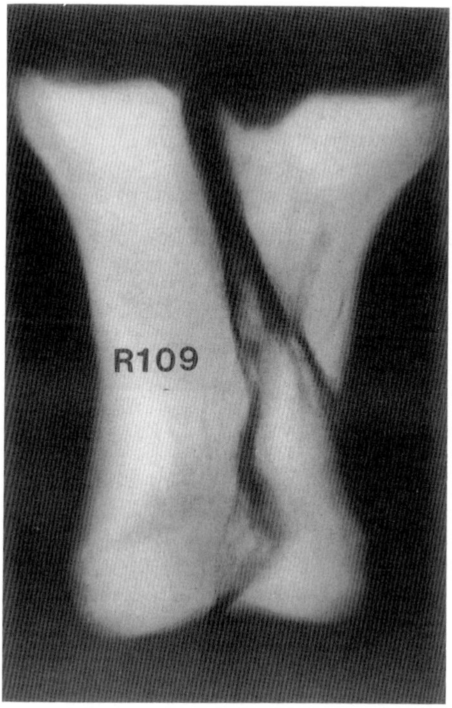

Fig. 155. Same horse as in Fig. 152. This is a radiograph of the right front long pastern bone seen from back. There is a comminuted fracture involving both ends.

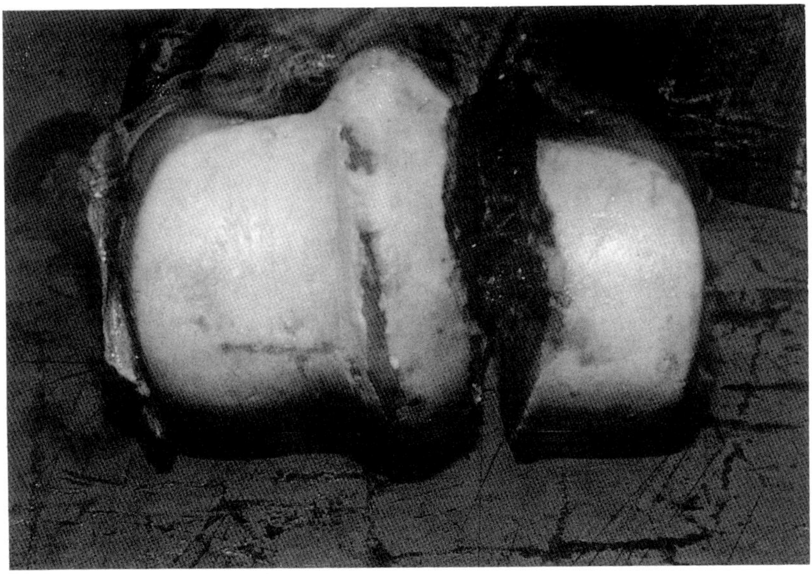

Fig. 156. Same horse as in Fig. 152. Lower end of right front cannon bone seen from back. The fracture separates the outer condyle. Note CON changes especially of the crest between the condyles.

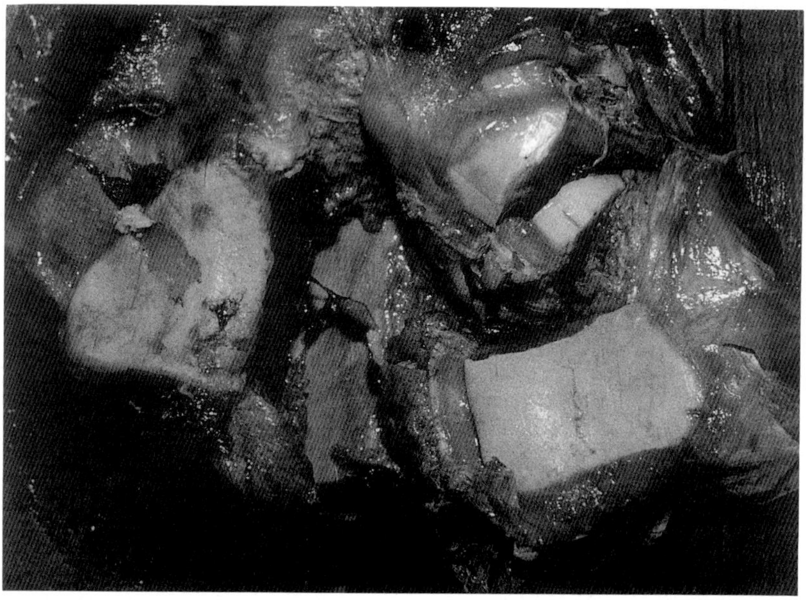

Fig. 157. Same horse as in Fig. 153. Sesamoid bones of right front limb seen from front. There is a comminuted fracture of the inner sesamoid bone (right). There is moderate destruction of the joint cartilage of the inner sesamoid bone and severe destruction of the outer bone. Note the cartilage damage of the lower inner part of the outer sesamoid bone, this is not a result of fracture but a pre-existing change.

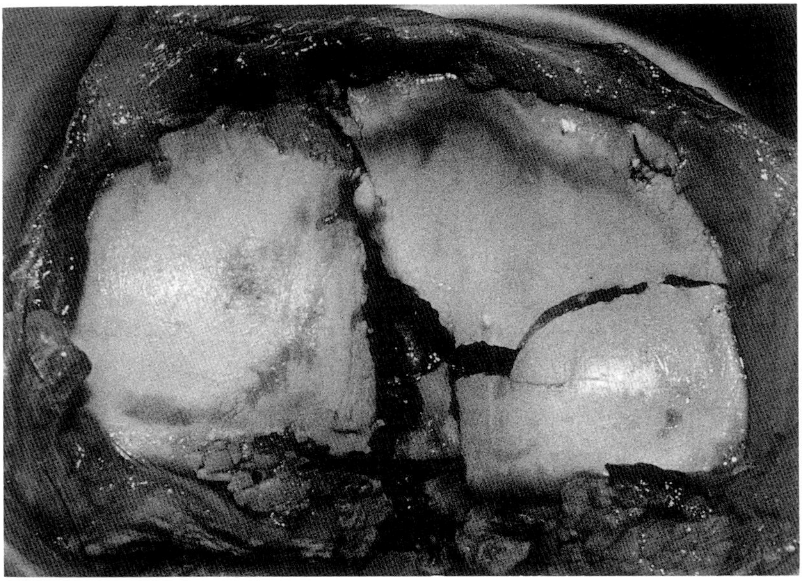

Fig. 158. Same horse as in Fig. 153. The upper end of the right front long pastern bone shows a comminuted fracture and severe CON changes. Note especially the back end of the inner condyle.

joint, extensive CON changes were present and confirmed by microscopic examination.

In this case, there is no way to explain the triple fracture by trauma. The fractures involved the three bones of the fetlock joint and all bones showed CON changes. The horse was terminated, not because of the stress of racing or training but, because of a primary disease of the three bones fractured. This disease was localized to the three bones forming the fetlock joint, all of which fractured. No similar changes were found elsewhere. The changes recorded are highly suggestive of corticosteroid injections into the fetlock joint.

REFERENCES

1. Jeffcott, K.B., S.E. Kold and F. Melsen. 1983. Aspects of the pathology of stifle bone cysts in the horse. Equine Vet. J. *15*:303-311.
2. Verschotte, F. and A. De Moor. 1982. Subchondral cystic and related lesions affecting the equine pedal bone and stifle. Equine vet. J. *14*:47-54.

VIII. PUTTING THINGS TOGETHER

1. Fractures in thoroughbred horses are pathologic, not traumatic.

Fractures in thoroughbred race horses are usually considered traumatic, and an unfavorable track condition is blamed. There are no statistical data to support this view. Further no one has come up with a definition or an unfavorable track condition. Is a fast track better or worse than off tracks (good, muddy, and sloppy)? As reviewed in Chapter VI, we analyzed the influence of track condition in 68,397 starts in flat races of thoroughbred race horses (12). We found that race track condition did not influence racing injuries in flat races of thoroughbreds. Consequently, we could not identify an unfavorable track condition. Thus, we discarded the concept that fractures in thoroughbred race horses in flat races are traumatic. All horses during a given race are exposed to the same track condition and the same stress of racing, and they are at the same traumatic risk. If bone fatigue (22,23) were of importance in the occurrence of fractures, then the fractures should occur mostly toward the end of a race and should increase with increasing distance of race, but they do not. Fractures occur at the start, the end, and anywhere during a race. The fracture incidence does not increase with increasing distance (12). The last case in the preceding chapter concerned a 4-year-old thoroughbred colt which fractured the right front cannon bone, a sesamoid bone, and the long pastern bone during a light workout, not a race. The fractures occurred not because of any trauma but because of pre-existing disease.

We must emphasize that our fracture material concerned thoroughbred horses during races. In this material, trauma cannot be considered a cause, only a triggering factor. We have no material from hurdle and steeple-chase racing. In such races, the horses are exposed to more trauma. We have no information on this subject in New York horses, but will briefly review a British report "A Clinico-Pathological Study on Racing Accidents in Horses" by Vaughan and Mason (26). Thoroughbred racing in Great Britain is very different from that in New York. Flat races constitute about 50 percent of all races and 50 percent are hurdle and steeplechase racing. The British study covered 34 months of flat racing and 29 months of all racing, including jumping races. The report stated that, in 1972, there were 26,495 starts in flat races and 25,409 in jumping races. When these figures are used for the entire study period, there would be about 75,000 starts in flat races and about 61,000 starts in jumping races.

The fractures incurred during races in the above-mentioned period are listed in Table 10. We have excluded from the 125 fatal accidents, dislocations of joints, pelvic fractures, fractures during training, and others. Table 10 tells, with adjustment for more starts in flat races, that the incidence of fractures during jumping races is about 6 times that in flat races. Fractures of back bones, all in jumping races, account for 17 percent of all fractures. The fractures during jumping races are, certainly, directly related to trauma.

Table 10. Distribution of fractures (Vaughan and Mason)

Bone fractured	Flat	Hurdle	Steeple-chasing
Back bones			
Neck	0	7	7
Chest-Loin	0	5	10
Front limbs			
Shoulderblade	1	1	3
Arm bone	0	2	6
Forearm bones	2	6	1
Knee bones	0	8	0
Cannon bone	3	4	3
Sesamoid bones	0	1	2
Long pastern bone	5	4	0
Hind limbs			
Thigh bone	0	0	3
Tibia	2	1	4
Hock bones	0	1	1
Cannon bone	0	0	3
Long pastern bone	3	1	0
Total	16	41	43

The British report estimated that 50-60 percent of all fractures were actually reported. If therefore we double the number of fractures, we find that the incidence of fractures in flat races would be 32 in 75,000 starts, that is 4.3 fractures in 10,000 starts. In our New York material, however, we recorded an incidence of 19.6 fractures per 10,000 starts. That incidence is more than 4.6 times that in British flat races. Why?

In the British material, the age of the horses fracturing bones during flat races averaged 2.9 years, in New York 3.5 years. The average distance in British flat races was 1 1/4 mile; in New York 54 percent of the races were less than one mile. In British jumpers, on the other hand, the average age of horses suffering fractures was 6.5 years and the average distance of the races was 2¼ mile.

2. The diseases causing fractures

As described in Chapter VII, there are three underlying diseases causing fractures in thoroughbred horses in flat races in New York:

A. Osteochondrosis (OCH). This is a developmental disease which we define as a failure of cartilage to convert into bone.

B. Chondro-osteo-necrosis (CON). This is an acquired disease which starts in the joint cartilage and eventually involves the underlying bone.

C. Tendon degeneration (TD).

A. *Osteochondrosis*

a. The nature of the disease

We have defined the disease as developmental and have described its various manifestations in Chapters IV, V and VII. Included in these manifestations are not only the cartilage changes but also osteopetrosis (which means too much bone tissue per volume unit of bones). OCH means, again, failure of cartilage to convert into bone. The coexistence of OCH and osteopetrosis may seem contradictory, but it is not. The bone tissue once formed before OCH came into the picture responds to the same thing that caused OCH, but responds in its own way. Normal removal of bone tissue is decreased, normal formation of bone remains normal, and the net result is too much bone tissue per volume unit of bones. We will return to this subject shortly.

The importance of OCH as a cause of fracture has been stressed in Chapter VII. Now comes the important question: What causes OCH? Since there is no first-hand information on this subject in horses, we will rely on information gained from studies in other species.

b. OCH in other species.

i. Bulls

A disease characterized by severe OCH, including OCD, and osteopetrosis was described in bulls (15,16). It was noted that the bulls had been overfed calcium, 3.5 times the recommended levels in young bulls and up to 6 times in older bulls.

ii. Dogs

Growing dogs of large breeds very often suffer from a variety of skeletal diseases that includes OCH and osteopetrosis. In a successful experimental reproduction of these diseases, weanling Great Dane puppies were fed a diet high in protein, energy and calcium. Calcium was fed at a level twice the recommended level (9). The puppies developed OCH, including OCD, and osteopetrosis. The findings were confirmed by a team in Holland (6,7,8). The Dutch researchers zeroed in on excessive dietary calcium with dietary protein and energy left at normal levels. Thus, excessive dietary calcium was established as the cause of OCH and osteopetrosis in dogs.

iii. Heifers

A farmer was advised by a feed company to feed heifers the same ration as given to milking cows. This turned out to provide more than 70 percent of calcium above the recommended level. The heifers developed severe skeletal disease, including OCH and osteopetrosis. A reversal to normal calcium feeding did not reverse the disease, but did prevent it in the next generation of heifers (24).

c. Nutritional hypercalcitoninism

Calcitonin is a hormone produced by the thyroid gland. Hypercalcitoninism means a state in which too much calcitonin is produced.

There are two hormones regulating the level of calcium in the blood: parathyroid hormone and calcitonin. Parathyroid hormone is produced by the parathyroid glands. The production of parathyroid hormone is stimulated by too low blood calcium, brought about, for instance, by too low dietary calcium. Parathyroid hormone acts on bone tissue to increase resorption, thus releasing calcium into the blood to compensate for the low blood calcium that caused the condition.

Calcitonin is the antagonist of parathormone. Calcitonin is produced in the thyroid gland by the C cells (C stands for calcitonin). The production is stimulated by high levels of calcium in the blood, hypercalcemia, and by high production of gastrin, a hormone manufactured in stomach and gut cells. Gastrin production is in direct proportion to the concentration of calcium in the stomach and gut. In excessive amounts calcitonin has two targets: cartilage and bone tissue. On cartilage, it reduces the normal maturation of cells and the conversion into bone, a process that is the very definition of OCH. On bone tissue, it reduces the rate of resorption without interfering with the rate of formation of bone. Thus, the net result is too much bone tissue per volume unit of bone, a state that is the very definition of osteopetrosis. In hypercalcitoninism, the reduced rate of resorption of bone tissue lowers blood calcium. The increased rate of gastrin production in response to high concentrations of calcium in the stomach and gut keeps hypercalcitoninism going in spite of lowered blood calcium.

Through the action of calcitonin, high dietary calcium will eventually lead to too low blood calcium. This stimulates the production of parathormone. Thus, in the long run, high dietary calcium will cause too high production of the antagonistic hormones calcitonin and parathormone. In this competitive state, the action on bone tissue by calcitonin overrules that by parathormone, and the osteopetrosis continues.

In summary:
i. Excessive dietary calcium causes
ii. Hypercalcemia and hypergastrinism, both of which cause
iii. Hypercalcitoninism. The targets for elevated calcitonin activity are
iv. Cartilage, where it reduces maturation of cells to cause OCH in all its variants, and bone, where it reduces resorption to cause osteopetrosis.

d. Calcium nutrition in the horse

i. Recommended dietary calcium levels

The National Research Council (NRC) published "Nutrient Requirements of Horses" in 1961 (17) and in 1978 (18). The recommended dietary calcium in grams per day were as follows:

	1961	1978
Nursing foal, 3 months of age, 340 lbs	17	33
Weanling, 6 months of age, 500 lbs	16	34
Yearling, 12 months of age, 715 lbs	13	31
Mature maintenance	12	23

For the 4 categories in the list, the 1978 recommendations in comparison to those of 1961 were increased by 94, 112, 138, and 92 percent, respectively. If the 1978 recommendations were right, then the 1961 levels certainly would have caused hyperparathyroidism ("big head"). There is no evidence that they ever did. On the contrary, if the 1961 recommendations were right, then the 1978 standards are high enough to cause hypercalcitoninism with its manifestations of OCH and osteopetrosis. We encounter plenty of these diseases in today's horses.

In foals with a mature weight of 1100 lbs., the nursing foal, 3 to 6 months of age, requires 33 grams of calcium per day. The mare provides 15 grams of calcium in the milk and NRC (18) therefore states that the "Requirement above milk" is 18 grams of calcium per day. In the opinion of NRC, the mare can provide only 45 percent of the calcium required by her foal. It seems that the very high "requirements" by NRC are at variance with Mother Nature.

In determining calcium requirements for horses, NRC (18) depended heavily on research in ponies. Data were then projected to horses. For a 2-year-old pony weighing 400 lbs. and a mature weight of 440 lbs., the requirement was stated to be 54 milligrams of calcium per 2.2 lbs. of bodyweight. For a 2-year-old horse weighing 1000 lbs. and a mature weight of 1100 lbs., the requirement was stated to be 55 milligrams per 2.2 lbs of bodyweight. Extending data from ponies to horses is a questionable approach. In general, a nutrient is required in inverse proportion to bodyweight. Data from NRC bulletins in the early 1960's were summarized (11) as follows: a 1400 lb. cow requires 17 milligrams of calcium per 2.2 lbs. of bodyweight; a 1400 lb. horse 20 milligrams; a 160 lb. sheep 52; a 110 lb. dog 62; a 22 lb. dog 95 and a 2.2 lb. dog requires 175 milligrams of calcium per 2.2 lbs. per day for mature maintenance. Thus, data obtained from 440 lb. ponies are hardly applicable to 1100 lb. horses.

ii. Feeding programs on horse farms

Osteochondrosis can occur in the newborn foal; in this case the changes are occurring in the fetal skeleton. When the pregnant mare is overfed calcium, she will produce higher than normal amounts of calcitonin. This does not hurt her own cartilage, since her skeleton is mature, not developing. Bone tissue is always formed and removed; this "turnover" of bone occurs in mature animals, though at a slower rate than in growing animals. Osteopetrosis can thus occur in the mare. Excessive calcitonin in the mare will be transmitted to the developing fetus. Since cartilage growth and bone turnover are very rapid in the fetus, the calcitonin action may have serious consequences.

Alfalfa hay contains about 6.6 grams of calcium per lb., timothy hay about 1.4 grams, sweet feed from 3.1 to 5.4 grams depending on brand, corn 0.1, and oats 0.7 grams of calcium per lb. It does not take many lbs. of alfalfa hay to exceed the recommended level of dietary calcium. Alfalfa is an excellent feed for high-yielding milking cows, but not for pregnant mares.

We have limited information on feeding programs at horse farms. We will give two examples how mares are fed according to information given by owners.

The feeds used at one very large standardbred farm are listed in Table 11. Alfalfa hay is the only roughage fed, and the mares consume very large amounts. Then sweet feed is added in more moderate amounts. These two sources provide from 7.4 to 10.2 times the recommended levels of dietary calcium. OCH is common among the foals.

At a thoroughbred farm with 22 mares, the mares are offered as much mixed hay (equal amounts of alfalfa and grass hay) as they want, and in addition, sweet feed at 15 lbs. per mare per day. This is together at least 130 grams of calcium per day. Then the mares are given dicalcium-phosphate in amounts not stated but that certainly add to the calcium excess.

Sweet feed is becoming very popular. It is a rich source of protein and energy that is needed by the mare. The very high concentration of calcium in sweet feed, from 0.7 to 1.2 percent varying with brands, is, however, not needed.

And how are the foals fed? The mare's milk provides enough calcium up to weaning. However, creep feed is offered first week or

Table 11. Feeding of mares at a standardbred farm in New York

Feed	Amount per day	Percent calcium	Calcium, grams
Alfalfa hay	30 - 40 lbs.	1.46	199 - 265
Sweet feed	2.2 - 3.3 lbs. per 220 lbs. bodyweight	1.08	54 - 81
Total			253 - 346
Times recommended levels			7.4 - 10.2

second week or "as soon as possible." One owner reported that from 9 to 15 lbs. of sweet feed was consumed by foals and 10 lbs. by yearlings. Another owner said that foals consumed the offered amount of 8 lbs. sweet feed and yearlings consumed as much as they wanted. The foals are overloaded with protein and energy so that they grow to an impressive size by the time of the yearling sales. The faster they grow, the higher is the activity in cartilage and bone tissue. The fast growth by itself does not cause OCH or osteopetrosis, but fast growth of cartilage and bone tissue makes these structures susceptible to dietary calcium excess.

B. *Condro-osteo-necrosis*

Chondro-osteo-necrosis (CON) means death of cartilage and bone tissue. The changes start in the joint surface cartilage, move deeper, and finally involve the underlying bone.

It is known that CON changes can develop within weeks or months after systemic injections (into muscles) of corticosteroids into horses (4,5). It has further been shown that a single injection into joints in horses caused CON changes that progress with time; once established, there is no healing (1). We have described and illustrated CON in a horse known to have had repeated injection of corticosteroids into a knee (Chapter VII, Figs. 66-68). In this case, the knee bones did not fracture, but the horse was disposed of because of severe lameness. In seven cases with knee bone fractures, the gross and microscopic changes in cartilage and bone (Figs. 103-107) were closely similar to those in the case of known chronic exposure to corticosteroids. Injection of corticosteroids as a common cause of these 7 knee fractures must be seriously considered.

Injection of corticosteroids for treatment of joint inflammation was first described in man in 1949 (10) and in 1951 (13). The first reference to such treatment in horses is from 1955 (27). The treatment has become widespread in horse practice to treat inflammation and pain, in spite of undesirable side effects.

In 1957 it was reported (21) that large doses of steroids taken by mouth in man caused death of joint cartilage, and those findings have been repeatedly confirmed (25).

In 1968, O'Connor (20) stated, in his paper "The untoward effects of the corticosteroids in equine practice," "Intra-articular injection [injection into a joint] of corticosteroids into horses with minor joint lesions produced immediate symptomatic relief, which encourages a damaging level of performance by interference with the normal protective mechanisms of simple inflammation. In time, as pain returns and the affected joint is reinjected, an endless destructive cycle is set into motion which, if continued, will produce a steroid arthropathy (joint disease) which can render the horse useless." (Words within [ ] are added). This timely warning was largely ignored. As noted above, the "endless destructive cycle" can be set into motion by one single injection (1).

In the collection of our fracture material, we were not privileged with information on previous treatments with corticosteroids. Thus we do not *know* the cause of the CON changes in the horses. It is noteworthy that these changes underlying fractures were observed in knee bones, at the ends of the cannon bone, and at the upper end of the long pastern bone. These are the bones that form the knee joints and the fetlock joint. These joints are exactly those where corticosteroid injections are commonly applied.

The widespread use of corticosteroids in horses is substantiated by data in "Annual Health Institute Annual Report 1985" (119 Oronoco St., Box 1417-D50, Alexandria, VA). In 1984, at least $3 million worth of corticosteroids for use in horses were manufactured in the US. This is the manufacturers' price. The price is increased in wholesale and retail distribution. Treatment of horses with corticosteroids is a multimillion dollar business.

C. *Tendon degeneration*

In fractures of the shaft of the cannon bone without involvement of either end and in fractures of the sesamoid bones, there were no changes in the joint cartilage or associated bone tissue to explain the fractures. Instead, the flexor tendons and the suspensory ligament, especially the branches toward each sesamoid bone, were consistently damaged. The changes included acute degeneration of tendon fibers with or without hemorrhages, mineral deposits in the damaged fibers, scar tissue formation, and a change of the tendon fiber cell into cartilage cells and even into bone-forming cells. Tendons so damaged lose their normal function, and pathological mechanical forces are acting on the cannon bone, the sesamoid bones (which are embedded in the suspensory ligament), on the pastern bones, and on the coffin bone.

The initial change is degeneration of the tendon fibers, with or without hemorrhages. The other changes are secondary, but more devastating to the tendon. The primary question is what caused the degeneration. Could it be the stress of training or racing? We do not believe so, because in that event there would be rupture of the fibers, which we have not observed. Further, the response to a traumatic rupture would not involve mineral deposits. We believe that the original damage to the tendon or ligament fibers is caused by injection of corticosteroids.

It has been shown that injection of corticosteroids into tendons of monkeys causes death of tendon cells (19), just as injection of corticosteroids into joints causes death of cartilage cells (reviewed above). The knee joint ligaments of the monkeys showed a 40 percent decrease in loading strength 6 to 15 months after the third injection when compared to non-injected control animals.

The effects on tendons and ligament by corticosteroid treatment have been documented in man. In one case (2), a male was treated systematically (route not stated) with the corticosteroid Triamcinolone for 5 months for a skin condition (Lupus erythematosus). He ruptured both Achilles tendons.

We now make reference to a case in which corticosteroids (hydrocortisone) were infiltrated into a ligament (14). A 25-year-old high jumper was treated for tenderness of the left knee (knee in man is the stifle in horses) with injections into the left knee ligaments. "This gave considerable relief, but the pain returned and persisted in milder degree, becoming worse when he was training." One month later, the ligaments were injected with "Triamcinolone." Relief of pain was temporary, but he continued jumping. He was seen again the next year with the same complaints. Ten months after the original treatment, the ligaments were injected twice with a 12-day interval with the same drug. Three months later, during a training session, he cleared 6′½″ and was attempting 6′2½″ when the accident occurred. "He had planted his left foot for take off at the end of the run and was on the point of lifting his right leg when the left foot slipped. He felt something give in his left knee and fell on his buttock. He had severe pain and was unable to get up or extend his knee." The left knee ligaments had ruptured.

Back to the horses. We have described and illustrated tendon degeneration (Figs. 69-81). The initial change is a degeneration of tendon fibers, which sets into motion reparative changes which eventually render the tendon non-functional. The acute changes are closely similar to those reported in experimental studies in other species (see above) as a result of corticosteroid exposure. We assume the same cause in horses.

Again, we have no information on the practice of injecting corticosteroids into tendons of horses. We do know that excessive dietary Vitamin D, another steroid, causes changes in tendons (Figs. 82 and 83) closely similar to those encountered in our fracture material. The response to one steroid is expected to be the same as that to another.

Using computer library search, we have not been able to find any descriptions of the microscopic damage to horse tendons and ligaments injected with corticosteroids. In a report on the results of injections of corticosteroids *around* tendons, including the suspensory ligament, and joints in standardbred horses, some devastating consequences were recorded (3). Corticosteroids, usually prednisolone, were injected twice at 100 milligrams around the inflamed structures. In one case, 8 injections were made over 15 months. Formation of bone tissue around the injection sites occurred within 4 to 11 months to a degree where it could be detected by manual inspection. The nature of the changes was verified by radiographic and microscopic examinations. It was further noted that, once started, the formation of bone tissue at the injection site grew worse even after withdrawal of the corticosteroid injections. In one case, the radiographically-diagnosed bone formation measured 1.2 by 0.2 inches 5 months after injections and 1.8 by 1 inch a little more than one year later.

Needless to say, such changes cause lameness, which is superimposed on the original cause of the lameness that the corticosteroid injections were supposed to cure. A short-lived, temporary relief of the clinical signs eventually resulted in aggravation of the condition. The author (3) concluded, in a remarkable understatement, that injections of corticosteroids around tendons, ligaments, and joints "should be avoided."

In the same vein, 4 years later, in 1969, Sweetnam (25) wrote in his editorial "Corticosteroid Arthropathy and Tendon Rupture": "We now have evidence, both clinical and experimental, that apart from the well recognized hazard of infection, intra-articular injections [injections into joints] of corticosteroids, certainly if repeated, may be harmful. It is also likely that the infiltration of corticosteroid around painful tendons in athletes, who are thereby enabled to continue their strenuous pursuits, may lead to tendon rupture. Until further evidence is forthcoming, therefore, it seems that the balance of evidence is in favor of the view expressed by Bentley and Goodfellow when they state that 'the case against multiple injections is so strong that the practice should, in our opinion, be discarded, which implies that even a single injection requires strong justification.' Likewise, corticosteroid injections around painful tendons in athletes should be discouraged because of the risk of rupture, particularly if the tendon is to be subjected to continued strain. Certainly no such injection should be given to an athlete without explanation of the risk involved." (Words within [ ] have been added).

3. The combination of osteochondrosis and chondro-osteo-necrosis

The combination of OCH and CON is, obviously, a very dangerous one. Each entity can cause fracture, and together they are devastating. Why do they occur together?

We will now describe an actual case, but we will restrict the details so that the case cannot be identified. A 3-year-old thoroughbred filly had a "handful of chips in her knees" (trainer's evaluation). This condition is, in our opinion, as documented in pictures in Chapter VII, an expression of OCH. These chips in the knee caused lameness on which the filly could not run. There was swelling and pain of the knee, both signs of an inflammation. The filly became a "basket case" with very little chance of future success. The affected knee was injected with corticosteroids (Depo-Medrol) 3 times over 70 days, the last time 2 days before a cheap claiming race. Shortly after the start, she fractured the cannon bone (whether knee bones were also fractured was never established because of a less-than-satisfactory post-mortem examination). The filly fell into two oncoming horses, which fell on their necks and were destroyed, as was the filly. Riding one of the oncoming horses was a jockey who sustained severe head injuries and became incapacitated for life.

This scenario, with a fatal outcome to the horse but not the jockey, is often repeated in thoroughbred races. OCH is a very common affliction of race horses that can and does cause chips in various joints. This sets up an inflammatory reaction, a cardinal sign of which is pain. This pain tells the horse not to run on an inflamed tendon or ligament or a joint. A horse cannot and should not train or race with any of these conditions. Then, however, corticosteroids are injected. They are powerful anti-inflammatory agents and, by blocking varying enzymes involved in the inflammatory process, extinguish the signs of inflammation, including pain. The horse is then led to the parade where it is declared racing sound because the signs of inflammation have been canceled by injection of a disease-inducing drug. We quoted above from Sweetnam (25): "Certainly no such injection should be given to an athlete without adequate explanation of the risk involved." The risk involved is not explained to the horse, which is not treated as an athlete but as a running machine expected to run just another race at the risk of his/her life. Nor is it explained to the horse's jockey or to the jockeys of other horses, all of whom run an increased risk of being injured by the fall of a horse treated with corticosteroids.

4. The bottom line

In this book we have presented the following facts and theories on breakdowns in thoroughbred race horses from New York race tracks.

A. *Facts*

a. Track condition has no influence on breakdowns, including fractures;

b. Fractures are pathological, not traumatic;

c. The underlying diseases leading to fractures are

i. Osteochondrosis, defined as a failure of cartilage to convert into bone;

ii. Chondro-osteo-necrosis, defined as a disease of the joint cartilage leading to death of cartilage and, eventually, of the underlying bone;

iii. Tendon degeneration.

B. *Theories*

a. Osteochondrosis is caused by excessive feeding of calcium to the pregnant mare, which will develop hypercalcitoninism. The excessive calcitonin affects the bones of the developing fetus and results in osteochondrosis and osteopetrosis;

b. Overfeeding the foal with protein and energy results in fast growth, which makes the growing cartilage and bone tissue susceptible to too high dietary calcium, which results in hypercalcitoninism;

c. Chondro-osteo-necrosis and tendon degeneration are caused by injection of corticosteroids into joints and tendons, respectively.

C. *The bottom line*

The disease leading to fractures in thoroughbred race horses are man-made. They are not curable, but they are preventable.

REFERENCES

1. Chunekamrai, S., L.P. Krook, G. Lust and G.A. Maylin, 1989. Changes in articular cartilage after injection of methylprednisolone acetate into equine joints. Amer. J. vet. Res. In press.
2. Cowan, M.A. and S. Alexander. 1961. Simultaneous bilateral rupture of Achilles tendons due to Triamcinolone. Brit. med. J. *1:*1658.
3. Garmer, L. 1965. Benmetaplasi, en komplikation till lokal terapi med corticosteroider hos häst (Osseous metaplasia, a complication to local corticosteroid treatment in the horse). Nord. Vet. Med. *17:*516-529.
4. Glade, M.J. and L. Krook. 1982. Glucocorticoid-induced inhibition of osteolysis and the development of osteonpetrosis, osteonecrosis and osteoporosis. Cornell Vet. *72:*76-91.
5. Glade, M.J., L. Krook, H.F. Schryver and H.F. Hintz. 1983. Morphologic and biochemical changes in cartilage of foals treated with dexamethasone. Cornell Vet. *73:*170-182.
6. Goedesgebuure, S.A. and H.A.W. Hazewinkel. 1986. Morphological findings in young dogs chronically fed a diet containing excess calcium. Vet. Path. *23:*594-605.

7. Hazewinkel, H.A.W. 1985. Influence of different calcium intakes on calcium metabolism and skeletal development in young Great Danes. Thesis. Utrecht, The Netherlands. Van den Berg's drukkerij b. v. Utrecht.
8. Hazewinkel, H.A.W., S.A. Goedesgebuure, P.W. Poulus and W.T.C. Wolvekamp. 1985. Influence of chronic calcium excess on skeletal development in growing Great Danes. J. Anim. Hosp. Assoc. *21:*377-391.
9. Hedhammar, Å, F.-M. Wu, L. Krook, H.F. Schryver, A. deLahunta, J.P. Whalen, F.A. Kallfelz, E.A. Nunez, H.R. Hintz, B.E. Sheffy and G.D. Ryan. 1974. Overnutrition and Skeletal Disease. An experimental study in growing Great Dane dogs. Cornell Vet. *64,* Suppl. 5:1-160.
10. Hench, P.A., E.C. Kendall, C.H. Slocumb and H.F. Polley. 1949. The effect of a hormone of the adrenal cortex (17-hydroxy-dehydro-11-dehydro corticosterone: Compound E) and the pituitary adrenocorticotropic hormone on rheumatoid arthritis. Proc. Mayo Clin. *24:*181-197.
11. Henrikson, P.-Å. 1968. Periodontal Disease and Calcium Deficiency. An experimental study in the dog. Acta Odontol. Scand. Suppl. *50:*1-132.
12. Hill, T., D. Carmichael, G. Maylin and L. Krook. 1986. Track condition and racing injuries in thoroughbred horses. Cornell Vet. *76:*361-379.
13. Hollandar, J.L., E.M. Brown, R.A. Jessar and C.Y. Brown. 1951. Hydrocortisone and cortisone injected into arthritic joints. J. Amer. med. Assoc. *39:*735-746.
14. Ismail, A.M., R. Balakrishnan and M.K. Rajakumr. 1969. Rupture and patellar ligament after steroid infiltration. J. Bone Jt Surg. *51B:*503-504.
15. Krook, L., L. Lutwak and K. McEntee. 1969. Dietary calcium, untimobranchial tumors and osteopetrosis in the bull. Syndrome of calcium excess. Amer. J. clin. Nutrition. *22:*115-119.
16. Krook, L., L. Lutwak, K. McEntee, P.-Å. Henrikson, R.K. Braun and S.J. Roberts. 1971. Nutritional hypercalcitoninism in bulls. Cornell Vet. *61:*625-639.
17. National Research Council. 1961. Nutrient Requirements of Horses. National Academy of Sciences. Washington, D.C.
18. National Research Council. 1978. Nutrient Requirements of Horses. 4th ed. National Academy of Sciences. Washington, D.C.
19. Noyes, R.F., N.S. Nussbaum, J.L. DeLuca and S.M. Cooper. 1975. Biomechanical and ultrastructural changes in ligaments and tendons after corticosteroid injection. J. Bone Jt Surg. *57A:*876.
20. O'Conner, J.T., Jr. 1968. The untoward effects of corticosteroids in equine practice. J. Amer. vet. med. Assoc. *153:*1614-1617.
21. Pietrogrande, V. and R. Mastromarine. 1957. Necrosis of articular cartilage following cortisone administration Ortop. Traumatol. app. Med. *26:*791-799.
22. Pratt, G.W. 1982. The response of high stressed bone in the racehorse. Proc. 28th Ann. Conv. Amer. Assoc. Equine Pract. Atlanta, GA. 31-37.
23. Pratt, G.W. and J.T. O'Connor. 1978. A relationship between gait and breakdown in the horse. Amer. J. vet. Res. *39:*249-253.
24. Rostkowski, C.M., T.D. Wilson, G.S. Allan, L.J. Deftos, K.W. Benson, F.A. Kallfelz, R.R. Minor and L. Krook. 1981. Hypercalcitoninism without hypercalcitoninemia. Cornell Vet. *71:*188-213.
25. Sweetnam, R. 1969. Editorial: Corticosteroid Arthropathy and Tendon Rupture. J. Bone Jt Surg. *51B:*397-398.
26. Vaughan, L.D. and B.J.E. Mason. 1975. A Clinico-Pathological Study of Racing Accidents in Horses. Adland & Son Ltd. Bartholomew Press, Doking, Surrey, U.K.
27. Wheat, J.D. 1955. The use of hydrocortisone in the treatment of joint and tendon disorders in large animals. J. Amer. vet. med. Assoc. *127:*64-67.

IX. VOCABULARY

Abduction. Latin abducere = to lead away. Turning outwards.
Acetabulum. Latin acetum = vinegar; acetabulum = vinegar cruet or vinegar crock. The acetabulum is the pelvic part of the hip joint.
Adduction. Latin adducere = to draw to one's self. Turning inwards.
Anatomy. Greek anatome = a dissection. The study of structure.
Antagonist. Greek antagonistes = competitor, opponent. For instance, calcitonin and parathyroid hormone are antagonists.
Arthrodia. Greek arthrodes = well jointed. A gliding joint between flat surfaces allowing only gliding movements.
Articulation. Latin = a joint.

-blast. Greek blastos = a germ, a forming cell. Osteoblast is a cell forming bone, etc.

Calcitonin. A hormone produced in the thyroid gland that decreases blood calcium.
Carpus. Greek karpos = a wrist. Carpus in horses is the knee.
Carpal bones—knee bones. There are two rows, upper and lower. In the upper row, the bones are from laterally: accessory, ulnar, intermediate and radial. In the lower row: 4th, 3rd and 2nd.
Cartilage. Latin cartilago, akin to cratis = a wickerwork. A translucent tissue that composes most of the skeleton in the embryo. Cartilage persists as the capping of the ends of bones.
Caudal. Latin cauda = a tail. Seen from behind; toward the tail.
Chondro-. Greek chondros = cartilage. Pertaining to cartilage.
Chondroblast. A cell forming cartilage.
Chondro-osteo-necrosis. Death of cartilage and bone, in that order. Abbreviated CON.
Circumdiction. Latin circumducere = to lead around. The circular movement of a limb.
Coccygeal. Greek kokkyx = cuckoo. The tailbone in man is said to resemble the bill of the cuckoo. Coccygeal = pertaining to the tail.
Collagen. Greek kolla = glue + gennan = to produce. The protein of connective tissues including bone, cartilage, tendon and skin.
Comminuted fracture. Latin comminutis, from con = together + minuere = to diminish. A shattered fracture.

Compound fracture. Latin componere = to put together. An open fracture through the skin.
Condyle. Greek kondylos = knuckle. A rounded projection of a bone for articulation with another.
Cortex. Latin = bark, rind or shell. The shaft of a long bone, also called the diaphysis.
Corticosteroid. Any compound with activities similar to those of the hormones produced by the adrenal gland cortex. Hydrocortisone, prednisolone, dexamethasone, Depo-medrol. Used in veterinary medicine as anti-inflammatory agent, pain killer.
Coxal. Latin coxa = hip. Pertaining to the hip.
Cranial. Greek kranion = skull. Seen from in front, toward the skull.
Crest. Latin crista. A projection from a bone. The ventral crest of the loin vertebrae of a horse projects ventrally to form the attachment for the ventral longitudinal ligament.
Cyst. Greek kystis = a bladder. An enclosed space within a tissue or organ, usually filled with fluid or other material.

Deltoid. Greek deltoides = shaped as the Greek letter delta. The deltoid tuberosity is located on the lateral side of the upper third of the humerus.
Diaphysis. Greek dia = between, through, apart or across. The shaft of a long bone. It consists of compact bone.
Digit. Latin digitus = finger or toe. The digit of the horse includes the long and short pastern bones and the coffin bone.
Distal. Latin distans = distant, away. In a limb, downwards.
Dorsal. Latin dorsum = back. Toward the back. Upwards in animals walking on all four limbs.

Embryo. Greek en = in + bryein = to swell. The fertilized egg is an embryo during the first 8 weeks.
Enarthrosis. Greek en = in + arthrosis = joint. A ball-and-socket joint which allows movement in all directions.
Epicondyle. Greek epi = on or upon. Epicondyle is an eminence on a bone upon its condyle.
Epiphysis. Greek epi = on or upon. The end of a long bone including the growth plate.
Epiphysitis. Inflammation of the epiphysis.
Etiology. Greek aitia = the cause + -logy, Greek logos = word, reason. A word ending meaning the "study of which." Etiology = the study of the cause of a disease.
Extension. Latin extendere = to straighten out. To increase the angle between bones.

Femur. Latin = thigh. The thigh bone.
Fetus. Latin fetare = to fertilize. An embryo turns into a fetus 8 weeks after conception.

Fibula. Latin = a buckle. Leg bone. The small bone on the lateral aspect of the tibia.
Flexion. Latin flexio = a bending. To bend bones, to decrease the angle between bones.
Fossa. Latin = a ditch. A hollow or depressed area.
Fracture. Latin fractura from frangere = to break. Fracture means a break of a hard tissue: bone, cartilage, tooth.

Gastrin. Greek gaster = stomach. A hormone produced in the stomach and gut in response to high calcium content. Gastrin stimulates the production of calcitonin.
Ginglymus. Greek ginglymos = a hinge. A hinge joint allows movement in one plane: flexion and extension.

Hemorrhage. Greek haima = blood + rhegnynai = to burst forth. Hemorrhage = a bleeding.
Humerus. Latin = shoulder. Humerus is the arm bone.
Hyper. Greek = above. A word beginning indicating too much of what follows.
Hypercalcemia. Too high level of calcium in the blood.
Hypercalcitoninism. A condition in which higher than normal amounts of calcitonin are produced.
Hyperparathyroidism. A condition in which higher than normal amounts of parathyroid hormone are produced.
Hypo. Greek = under. A word beginning meaning too little of what follows.

Ilium. Latin. One of the three paired hip bones.
Inflammation. Latin inflammare = to set on fire. Inflammation means the localized response by body cells and fluids to an injury. "The true signs of inflammation are four: redness and swelling with heat and pain" (Celsus, 30 B.C.-38 A.D.). A fifth sign, loss of function, was added later (Galenus, 129-201). An inflammation of a tissue or ogran is indicated by the addition of the word ending -itis. See below.
Inter-. Latin = between. For instance, intercarpal = between carpal bones; between knee bones.
Intra-. Latin = within. For instance, intra-articular = within a joint.
Ischium. Greek ischion = hip. One of the three paired hip bones.
-ism. A word ending indicating a condition resulting or involving the preceding, usually composite noun. For instance, hypercalcitoninism means a condition in which too much calcitonin is operating in the body.
-itis. A word ending indicating an inflammation. For instance, osteitis is an inflammation of bone tissue.

Lateral. Latin latus = side. Seen from the outside; outwards.

Ligament. Latin ligare = to bind. A strong band of connective tissue that connects bones.
Longitudinal. Latin longitudo = length. Parallel to the long axis.

Malleolus. Latin malleus = a hammer; malleolus = a little hammer. The lateral malleolus of the tibia is a rounded prominence on the lateral side of the distal end of the tibia.
Matrix. Latin = a womb. The groundwork of the soft part of bone tissue.
Medial. Latin medial = middle. Seen from the midline; inwards.
Medullary space. Latin medulla = marrow. The marrow space within bones.
Metacarpus III. Greek meta = beyond, distal. The cannon bone of the front limb.
Metacarpus II and IV. The splint bones of the front limb.
Metaphysis. The part of a long bone beyond the growth plate. It consists of trabecular bone.
Metatarsus III. The cannon bone of the hind limb.
Metatarsus II and IV. The splint bones of the hind limb.
Mitosis. Greek mitos = a thread or a string which refers to the thread-like arrangement of cell components during cell division. Mitosis—cell division.
Morphology. Greek morphe = shape + -logy. The study of forms and structures.

Navicular bone. Latin navicula = a boat. The boat-shaped bone. Also called the distal sesamoid bone.
Necrosis. Greek nekros = a corpse. Necrosis means death of a tissue or an organ.
Nucleus. Latin nux = a nut; nucleus = a small nut, a kerbel, a pot, a stone. The nucleus is the growth center of a cell.
Nutrient foramen. Latin nutrire = to nourish + foramen = an opening. The opening in the shaft of a long bone for blood vessels.

Olecranon. Greek olene = elbow + kranion = skull. The skull of the elbow bone.
-osis. A word ending indicating a non-inflammatory process.
Ossification. Latin os = bone + fecare = to make. Formation of bone tissue.
Osteo-. Greek osteon = bone. Pertaining to bone. Osteoblast. A bone-forming.
Osteochondrosis (OCH). Greek osteo = bone + chondros = cartilage + osis. OCH means, literally, a non-inflammatory condition involving bone and cartilage. OCH is defined here as a failure of cartilage to convert into bone.
Osteochondrosis dissecans (OCD). Latin dissecare = to cut up. The separation of cartilage with or without a piece of bone from the main structure.

Osteopetrosis. Greek osteo = bone + petra = a stone. Too much bone tissue per volume bone: "rock solid bone."

Parathyroid hormone. A hormone produced in the parathyroid glands that causes resorption of bone which results in increased blood calcium.

Patella. Latin patera = a shallow dish; patella = a small shallow dish. Patella is the knee cap.

Pathology. Greek pathos = disease. The study of diseases.

Pathologic. Indicative or caused by a disease process.

Pelvis. Latin = a basin. The bony ring formed by three paired bones (the ilium, ischium, the pubis), the sacrum and the first 3 coccygeal vertebrae.

Peri-. Greek = around.

Perichondrium. The membrane around the cartilage.

Periosteum. The membrane around bone.

Phalanx. Greek = a line or array of soldiers. The 1st phalanx or P I is the long pastern bone, the 2nd phalanx or P II is the short pastern bone, the 3rd phalanx or P III is the coffin bone.

Physis. Greek phyein = to generate. The growth plate which is situated inside either or both ends of a long bone and from which longitudinal growth occurs.

Process. Latin. A prominence or a projection on a bone.

Proximal. Latin proximus = nearest. In a limb = upwards.

Pubis. Latin. One of the three paired hip bones.

Radius. Latin = spoke or rod. The forearm bone.

Rotation. Latin rotare = to turn. Turning around an axis.

Rupture. Latin rumpere = to break. Rupture is a tear of soft tissues such as tendons and ligaments. Compare fracture.

Sacrum. Latin = sacred. One of the pelvic bones.

Scapula. Latin = shoulder. The shoulder blade.

Sesamoid bone. Greek sesame = sesame. Sesamoid = shaped like a sesame seed. Sesamoid bones are embedded in tendons. The proximal sesamoid bones are located on the back side of the fetlock.

Skeleton. Greek skeltos = dried up. The bony framework of the body.

Spicule. Latin spiculum = A small spike-shaped bone.

Sub-. Latin sub = under, beneath. For instance, subchondral means beneath the cartilage.

Suspensory ligament. Latin sus = up + pendere = to hang down. Latin ligare = to bind; ligament = a bandage. A strong bandage that connects bones. The suspensory ligament is a highly modified muscle, mostly tendinous.

Talus. Latin = ankle.

Tarsus. Greek tarsos = "a frame of wickerwork." Ankle or hock.

Tendon. Latin tendere = to stretch. The end of a muscle which attaches to a bone.

Tibia. Latin = a pipe, flute. The main leg bone.
Trabecula. Latin trabs = a beam; trabecula = a little beam. A bone spicule.
Transverse trabeculae. Latin transversus, from versus = to turn; transversus = crosswise. The arrangement of bone spicules parallel to the joint cartilage or the growth plate, as opposed to the normal perpendicular arrangement.
Trauma. Greek = wound or injury. An injury caused by a mechanical or physical agent.
Trochanter. Greek trachein = to run. The greater trochanter of the femur is a large process on the lateral, proximal end. The lesser trochanter is on the medial side.
Tuber calcanei. Greek tuber = a hump; tubercle = a little hump. The great tubercle of the humerus is located on the lateral side of the upper end.

Ulna. Greek olene = elbow. The elbow bone.

Ventral. Latin venter = a belly. Toward the belly. Downwards in animals that walk on all four limbs.
Vertebra. Latin vertere = to turn. A back bone.
Vesicle. Latin vesica = a blister; vesicula = a little blister.

IX. ACKNOWLEDGEMENTS

Figs. 1-10 are reproduced from "An Atlas of Animal Anatomy for Artists" by W. Ellenberger, H. Baum and H. Dittrich, second edition, edited by L.S. Brown and published in 1956 by Dover Publications, Inc., 180 Varick Street, New York, NY, 10014. We thank the publisher for courteous permission to reproduce these illustrations.

Many of the illustrations in this book have been previously published in THE CORNELL VETERINARIAN (Figs. 11-17, 23, 24, 29, 47, 66-81, 84-101, 103, 106-108, and 110-152). We appreciate the permission to reproduce these pictures.

Figs. 18-22, 25-28, 48-63, 82, 83, 102, 104, 105, 109 and 153-158 are new, never published before.

We thank Anne Krook, Ph.D., Department of English, College of Arts and Sciences, Cornell University, for editorial assistance.